# About the Author and Editor

Keith Terry has been writing for several decades. He lives with his wife, Ann, in Provo, Utah.

Wesley B. Jarvis is a lifelong researcher into Book of Mormon prophecy. He has found areas of vital interest in documentation and revelation that have thus far eluded many in the LDS community. Even its assiduous scholars have not yet perceived or written about some of these well-camouflaged materials. Among these are scriptures that are positive about Nephite preservation and identification.

Now retired from years of welding at the Geneva Steel Plant in Utah, he has been an active member of the Church and a temple worker. Twice widowed, he is married to his third lovely wife, Josephine. They make their home in Orem, Utah.

# The Greater Things

By

# Keith Terry
# Wesley Jarvis

*First published by VAD*
*Second Printing BeeJay Publishing*
*Copyright © Wesley Jarvis and Keith Terry*

ISBN 0–9668360–0–6

Printed in the United States of America

# Acknowledgments

Our sincere thanks to Josephine Jarvis, Jerry St. Vincent, and Ann Terry for their help with this project. Also, it is a special thanks that we give to Ferrin and Martha Whittaker for their support in this project.

# Dedicated to

Ferrin and Martha Whittaker

# Chapter 1

CNN's Tom Carey, assistant editor, Jerusalem bureau, held the portable mike as close to Morris Herschner, the Temple Committee chairperson, as he could possibly reach from the side of the field recorder that his cameraman was shoving in the face of this Jewish spokesperson.

At a slight distance, Samuel and Brad Meyers—grandfather and grandson, ages 73 and 23— stood transfixed on the edge of the cluster of newspeople who had swarmed around Herschner, a longtime friend of Samuel Meyers. Cameras everywhere whirred to capture on tape the unfolding events of the moment. The word had spread that the Jewish hierarchy had a monumental announcement concerning the Temple site in the Old City. The whole media corps turned out; they even flew in from Europe and the United States to cover the story. All they knew for certain was that the powers that be in the orthodox Jewish community were to announce the first step in rebuilding the ancient Temple of Solomon. That announcement alone was enough to bring to the foot of the Dome of the Rock the usually staid press corps in Jerusalem.

Samuel had to pull back on being so mentally critical of the media. His own tall, lean, bleached-blond grandson Brad was now twenty feet in front of Samuel, elbowing his way to the front of the crowd like a pro.

Brad had accompanied his grandfather on this latest jaunt to the Holy Land. "My boy," the admiring grandfather had requested, "I don't want to impinge on your schooling, but I have a deal: Can you accompany me on a couple of trips and do some of the basic filming for a video I'm involved in concerning the coming of the Millennium?" Brad had leapt at the opportunity. He even got the professor in his UCLA film class to give him credit for the semester while he took time off from regular class activity to join his grandfather. "Is it a deal?" Samuel had asked. "A deal, Gramps," Brad had replied, figuring he was his grandfather's favorite (which was typical of the way each of Samuel's fifteen grandchildren felt). He was that kind of grandfather, had been that sort of dad, and though a widower now, he had treated his late wife, Margaret, in like fashion. She always felt while married to Samuel that she was the most special person in the world to him.

A hundred feet to the north, where Herschner was now pointing for the benefit of the news hounds, were cream-colored, rust-veined, Jerusalem stone blocks, hewn anciently out of surrounding cliffs, the size of microwave ovens. Who knew exactly where or when they had been placed in formation? The stones constituted the foundation of a flat stone floor that extended to the east wall of the Old City—the Golden Gates—where the eastern gates would be opened one day to allow the Messiah to enter.

With growing excitement, Samuel watched as the several news video cameras and correspondents with hand-held Canons, Yashikas, and Nikons focused on the location that Morris Herschner had just declared to be the exact spot where the ancient Temple of Solomon rose. "The domain is over there. Yeah, right over there. That's it," Herschner repeated. "No question about it. The site has been measured, drilled, slightly excavated, and compared with the ancient writings of Yechetzqyah (the Prophet Ezekiel), who took the time anciently to record, in minute detail, the temple site."

It was clear to all present that the crescent bags under Herschner's eye lids revealed a man who had experienced travail in his lifetime. He was small boned and narrow faced, with the gray, well-wrinkled, facial skin characteristic of a person in his late seventies. He had arrived in Jerusalem shortly after the ' 67 war and took a position at the University of Jerusalem, which now stood on the northeast hills from the Old City.

With a small, hand-held mike in his left hand, Herschner took a sheet of paper from his black plastic folder and held it close to the reading glasses perched on the bridge of his long, narrow nose and said, "This spot where you see the Dome of the Rock has been a great contention between Jews and Moslems. Today, a grand new   understanding of revelation now offers a peaceful solution.

"Found in the Biblical record, which is called Ezekiel by the Christians but whom we call Yechetzqyah, is a plan and place for the  new temple to be erected, and the great news I offer you is that the plans do not involve the Dome of the Rock!" Morris paused long enough to let his words take effect on those listening. "Needless to say this is earth-shaking news, and I will now show to you exactly where this great temple, according to revelation, will be raised. After much study, measuring, and intense discussion, we have determined that the Dome of the Rock was constructed in the former south courtyard of the ancient temple."

There was a buzz of excitement set off among those gathered. This was news.

Samuel stood back, able to hear every word Herschner spoke into the portable mike. As he listened for more, it crossed his mind that one vital fact of the great sacrifice of Abraham was lacking. Morris had, of course, not spoken of the symbolic sacrifice of Isaac as a type of the atonement of Jesus Christ in which God the Father would sacrifice His Only Begotten Son for the salvation of all mankind. Someday the Jews and Moslems would come to realize this fact, but not yet.

Herschner continued to read from the sheet a statement he had prepared and had submitted to the reigning Jewish authority the day before. He asked that media people, who made up the bulk of his audience, allow him to read his statement that had the stamp of approval from the Jewish ecclesiastic authority. He didn't expect an answer from the hardened expressions immediately in front and to the side of him. "I will be free to answer any question as soon as I have read this important statement. Okay?

"I begin by flatly stating that in Yechetzqyah's prophecies are the complete measurements of a temple—a temple unlike any other that has ever been built before."

Samuel listened attentively, his right ear turned slightly in order to make audio contact with every word Herschner read from his statement. Herschner's voice carried well in the open plaza as he spoke into the Radio Shack microphone.

"Many of these measurements in the Bible have never made sense to scholars," Herschner said with a slight German accent in his delivery as he continued to read from the typed sheet, "but with Yahweh's inspiration we have come to see exactly what the Prophet Yechetzqyah saw in vision. We now are convinced, after our engineers have done exhaustive studies on the foundations of each area within the confines of where we had supposed the temple site stood, that it is clear that the Dome of the Rock does not stand on the actual temple site." The professor paused at this juncture. Then he found his place on the sheet and began reading again: "There is an absolutely amazing prophecy, a prophecy that Yechetzqyah was inspired by Yahweh to write. In this prophecy, he gives the measurements of the third and last Temple! These measurements have never been used before in the manner in which Yechetzqyah gave them. The first temple was built under Solomon; the second temple was rebuilt by Zerubbabel, which was later refurbished by King Herod. But, you may ask, what makes this prophecy amazing? I'll tell you. It reveals that Yechetzqyah saw the Temple Mount in vision in our day, with a building which sits upon it at the present time. I also wish to tell you that these temple measurements were inspired by Yahweh.

"Yechetzqyah shows us the Temple Mount as it appears in this day—not in his day. That is, when he was alive. In Ezekiel 40:1–5, we see that the measurements that he wrote are to be used now by this generation. Listen to what the prophet wrote in the scriptures: 'Then the being said to me, Son of man, look with your eyes and hear with your ears, and fix your mind upon everything that I show you; for the purpose that I show this to you, were you brought here. Declare all that you see to the House of Israel.' Verse five: 'And behold, there was an adjoined separation, a dividing structure, around a temple. In the being's hand was a measuring reed six cubits long—about ten and a half feet—each cubit about eighteen inches, with a handbreadth plus about three inches. So he measured the separation's width to the structure, one reed, about ten and a half feet; and height, rise, one reed. He did measure the Temple's foundation.'"

Herschner looked directly into the maze of cameras, and with sheer determination in his voice, Samuel and the others heard him make his pronouncement and plea, "Never before in this history of the Temple has the Temple been built *without* its outer court. But never before has there been a mosque sitting on the Temple Mount. As you see, the Dome of the Rock to my left is located over the Rock or Temple Mount." Herschner extended his arm and with his thin index finger he pointed up at the Arab world's shrine, the Dome of the Rock. "Interestingly, in this prophecy, the outer court is *not* rebuilt; apparently it is not required for the third Temple when erected. The temple will stand to the north, beside the Dome of the Rock Mosque, with only a dividing wall separating the Dome from the inner court. These measurements given by the prophet show that this dividing wall separating the mosque from the inner court serves no defensive purpose; it only serves as a privacy fence. Yahweh shows us that we do not need to retake the Arab's sacred site; we do not need to fight over the Temple Mount! Yahweh is showing us that we can and we should build this Temple on the vacant land where the Temple proper stood before, and that we should build a dividing wall to separate the Arab worshipers from the Jewish worshipers!

"I wish to add one other comment before I answer questions. This latest revelation from on high can be the salvation of Israel and Yahdah. We are facing a time when only a Super Power can save us, and prophecy shows us that this Super Power will save us—that is, if we act now by obeying the laws and fulfilling these simple prophecies." Herschner clapped his hands.

Brad was close enough at the moment to get the sound clearly as well as the image on his video recorder. He had worked his way to the very front and felt satisfied that he had a marvelous take of this dramatic moment.

"Now then, my friends, I am yours for the next while to answer any questions you may have."

At the edge of the jockeying crowd, Samuel, thrilled at the news reverberating through his system, realized that in all likelihood he might be the only one present who understood the full impact of what was being announced. It was one of the prophesied events to usher in the final days. It meant that in the near future the Jews could perhaps begin construction on the site over there and one day welcome the Savior as he was prophesied to descend out of the clouds of heaven, making his approach to the Jewish temple from the east. Amazing.

Samuel stepped two paces to the left to get a better view of exactly where Morris had pointed when he announced the original site of the temple.

Samuel knew the importance of such a find. He also was aware that to the Jews there was really only one temple. He understood, as a devoted student of the scriptures and the history of the Hebrews, that this was welcome news that would have a direct impact on the Jewish and Arab world. Actually, the discovery of a new site would be picked up by all the wire services, broadcast everywhere, and received with rejoicing and misgivings.

Tom Carey, a tall man with a rather awkward appearance, but a good news chief in the Near East, asked, "The temple site is farther over to the left. Is that what you are telling us? Are you saying that it does not interfere with the Dome of the Rock? And also, Dr. Herschner, are you also saying that your people, the Jews, in the near future are prepared to build your temple on that site?"

It took a moment for Morris to respond to Carey's question. "Yes, that is exactly what I think will happen. We have the funds available to build the temple."

Samuel knew that for at least a decade Morris had been associated with the Jewish Temple Architectural Committee, and that the professor was a vital link between the committee and the public. But this latest announcement—wow! Morris implying that there was a peaceful way to resolve the deadlock between Islam and the Jews over who had rights to what real estate and the influence to pull it off. Samuel reasoned that the Jews clearly had a scripture deed to build on the stone remains of the property to the north. Didn't they? But Samuel was realistic enough to know that there were hoops yet to jump through for the Jews before the rebuilding of the Jewish Temple became a reality. But they were on to something.

He had known of the day when the Jews would be inspired to rebuild their sacred temple since he first started studying the fate of the Jews in the scheme of things to come in a chain of events that would lead up to the Second Coming of Christ. Lately, he had devoted his life to a detailed search of the events to come. At 73 he had serious doubts whether he would have the stamina to withstand the grueling schedule he had designed for himself. But then Samuel had always possessed energy to do whatever task he put his mind to.

Samuel Meyers revealed physical features of his strong German genes in his every movement. Once blond, of medium height, a face almost too narrow, lines in the cheeks, bright deep-blue eyes with dark lashes and eyebrows. He was what anyone in the western world would consider a good-looking older man. At the moment he felt a little too warm in his forest-green wool pullover, but not terribly uncomfortable. After all, it *was* November, and even in this sunny Mediterranean climate it could get chilly if he were to stand in the shade. Still, it was a resplendent noon resembling his hometown, Boise, Idaho, in the spring.

Samuel pondered the setting and the moment of this momentous announcement he had heard. He longed to share it with his Katherine, who was, he thought, in Greece. He knew it would merely puzzle her. His deceased wife Margaret would have understood, but Katherine hadn't the scriptural background to appreciate the significance of it. Ah, well. At least Brad, whom Samuel could see making his way back to him, had been present to share the moment.

* * *

Sidney knocked and the door opened.

"Sid, Sid, thanks for coming," Samuel Meyers nearly shouted, throwing wide open the door to let his old friend enter the room. The two had remained close friends over more than twenty-five years. Samuel grabbed his large hand as the old friend spread a smile across his broad face. They hadn't seen each other for more than six months, but time was immaterial.

He came striding into the second-floor room at the St. David Hotel. In spite of his extra forty pounds, at sixty he moved like a man in his forties. Sidney Bender's wide facial features and large inquisitive eyes seemed to miss nothing. To Samuel, he looked refreshed; there was a tanned glow to his skin. The crow's feet around his brown eyes had white in the lines. He had been in the sun more than usual. With the look of his Irish ancestors, he possessed the demeanor of a doer. He had been at the head of Ancient Scripture at Brigham Young University for the past ten years. A few minutes ago he had taken leave from his tour group that was assembling in the lobby, preparing to go to Masada for the afternoon, to see his old friend Samuel Meyers, whom he had heard was also in Jerusalem, right here at the St. David. The hotel was still the watering hole for the well to do, located as it was between the Old City and downtown Jerusalem.

"I didn't know you were here in the city until last night when I saw your picture in the paper meeting with a group of scholars. Then, checking around, I come to find out you're right here in the St. David. What are you doing here?" Sid asked.

"Come in and have a seat." Samuel waved his hand in the direction of the sofa and coffee table on the far end of the room near the windows. "What am I doing here? I couldn't resist being on hand for the Jewish temple announce-ment —you know, the new site that the Jews plan to build on. I actually learned about the temple site just today. I'm gathering information on events that will take place in this city prior to the Second Coming." Samuel backed away to let Sidney step past him. "Anyway, I'm glad you've taken time out to pop in for a minute. I really want to talk with you. I just wish I weren't leaving so soon for Europe."

Bender lowered his overweight body to the sofa, exposing the top of a bald dome pink from too much sun. He sighed. "So do I. Why do you suppose we rush so much at our age? It's good to just sit for a while. I don't complain a whole lot, but I can't think of anything that taxes my strength like crawling around ruins. We were in Jericho this morning. The sun was too much. I think I'll just stay right here in this cool room and let you entertain me with your latest discoveries," he added with a smile. "This temple thing is exciting."

"You wish. You said that your group is visiting Masada this afternoon."

"You're right, but I can dream."

Samuel sat down on a white, hardwood chair across from Bender. "Why do you keep bringing tours here to the Holy Land if it's such a chore?"

"I love this part of the world. Also, it affords me time for ongoing research. I've made a few friends here at the universities. Besides, it's all paid."

"I see."

"I've heard about your latest project, and I want you to fill me in."

"Now?"

"No. But when we get back. I'll even come up to your place in Boise if you will just let me in on some of your research. I may teach religion, but not the coming of the Millennium. They say you are going all out on this thing about the Second Coming. Is that true?"

"I'm certainly putting in time, but there's no need for you to come up to Boise. I'll be in Provo most of the time working with Pete Polk on his Book of Mormon Center projects. We can just get together when we have a minute."

"You mean you moved from your home in Boise?"

"No. I still have the house, though it's not the same anymore. I miss her. Man, do I miss her."

"I think I know how it must be to lose someone dear to you."

It had been two years since Samuel lost his wife, and still at times the thought of her no longer around would come crashing in on him like an angry wave. It never got as easy as some insisted it would. Since Katherine had begun filling the void, she was closer to his heart than any other woman in his current life. The relationship with someone so tender and compassionate tended to ease the pain, and he found he thought of his deceased wife less and less often.

"Boy, I was really impressed with your report on the survival of a remnant of Nephites. Are you getting any static on that theory?" Bender wanted to know.

"Some," Samuel agreed. Bender knew he had other things on his mind at the moment and Bender sensed it when he said, "There is something I want to pick your brain about, Sam. I know you're not a professional scholar, though you've spent a good deal of time in books."

"Right, I've pursued the scriptures through the years as CEO of the lumber company. I've kept on probing those items of research that piqued my interest."

"Yes, I would have to say you did."

"As you seem to already know, I'm involved in this project that ties in with the events leading up to the Second Coming of the Savior."

"The Brethren have given you an assignment?"

"No. It's not that serious nor perhaps as important . . . well, it's important, but I accepted an assignment to ferret out information that will be useful to us in setting up a display in the Book of Mormon Center. I'm not setting myself up as some sage who has all the answers. I'm simply looking at the foretold events and documenting them."

"Just old simple researching, eh, Samuel?" There was a tinge of sarcasm in Bender's remark that was not lost on Samuel. "Tell me something: Have you had any static or backlash from anywhere about the Center and what you guys have done so far? You know, setting up a center and displaying the results of much of the research that has been done in the last decade?"

"No. Not at all. People seem to think it's a good idea to focus attention on the Book of Mormon. Still, it's a lot of work. But let me tell you, it has been exhilarating. It seems to consume a good deal of my time."

"Surely not all. I hear you've been seeing a lady these past few months. How does she feel about all of this?"

"Well, well, Sid, I see the religion department's grapevine hasn't wilted."

Sidney grinned. "Who is she?"

"Maria knows her. It was her ship we were on in the Pacific. Ask Maria."

"It was Maria who told me about her. What's her name? I already know she's from San Francisco."

"We met on her ship and were attracted to one another. Her name's Katherine Moore, and I find her one of the most charming ladies I've met in a long while."

"Sounds serious."

"I haven't asked her to marry me, if that's what you mean."

"Okay, I'll back off. Just curious. I understand she's got lots of money, though you haven't done too badly yourself. You people just don't spread it around, do you?"

"Come on, Sid, you're making a giant leap to a marriage that may not happen." Samuel rubbed his earlobe and let a slight grin cross his face.

"I didn't come up here to dabble in your love life. I want to know what you've uncovered that is not the usual stuff of Crowther and the other scribes of the prophecies leading up to the Second Coming. You've got to have something startling or it wouldn't be attracting *your* attention and taking up so much of your time."

"I don't know how startling it is, but I've been poking around here—"

"Meaning here," Bender pointed at the floor, "Jerusalem?"

"Yeah. As well as in parts of Asia and South America for the past couple of months. You know—just roaming around pulling together data. A lot of it has been the usual stuff: wars in the last days; famines, plagues, conflicts that are supposed to happen in the land; judgments; Armageddon; the New Jerusalem; Adam-ondi-Ahman; that sort of thing." Samuel stopped short of the complete list of events. With Bender long ago he had developed the habit of speaking in short hand. It was just the way they approached things of mutual interest. "What I'm doing is a kind of service to Pete Polk. The poor guy is having a devil of a time with his health."

"Yeah, when did you last see him? I heard that he was some athlete at Logan when you two were at school there. Now he's just a shell of the former man."

"He isn't an athlete anymore. He's in a wheelchair but very much alert. His doctor insists he not take on any additional work, so he asked me if I would follow up on this project he had on the boards for his Book of Mormon Center but couldn't get at. But he is anything but a shell."

"I thought that Center was all wrapped. Don't they already have a horde of tourists visiting it there in Provo?"

"Sure, but we want to expand it."

"We? When did you get that involved?"

"It's been over six months."

"I don't think I'll ever figure out just what makes you tick. Here you are, what? How old are you?"

"I'm 73, so treat your elders with respect."

"Okay, but my gosh, man, you deserve a little time on the golf course."

Samuel shook his head. "That's not me."

"Oh, well. Okay, so you're tracking down the events. Let me tell you something that I don't readily admit to, not to students anyway. I haven't really given a lot of time to prophecy leading up to the coming of the Savior. It's one area of my studies that is seriously lacking in understanding. I would be hard-pressed to give a series of lectures on the subject, or even one. Though I have to admit that lately I have more than a passing interest in studying the events that have to take place."

"Good, Sid. I ought to hire you as my assistant."

"You wouldn't be getting a very good deal. Besides, what does the Book of Mormon Center have to do with preparation for the Second Coming of Christ?"

"Plenty."

"Such as?"

"You know as well as anyone that the Lord spent a good deal of his time talking about events leading to his Coming when he visited the Nephites shortly after his resurrection."

"That's true."

" He did. He dwelt on the subject throughout his revelations in the Doctrine and Covenants and in his discourse to the Nephites. I suspect he said a great deal more than we've been given in Third Nephi about his Coming. They are likely sealed up in the plates Joseph Smith was not allowed to translate. At our Book of Mormon Center we want to present exactly what Christ said about his Coming. So, what better source than his own words out of the Book of Mormon? Of course there are other scriptures that mention it as well, and a lot of evidence in the earth. We want to display this very graphically in the Center."

"Okay. So tell me all about the Second Coming."

"Wow. Sid, it isn't that simple. We don't begin to have the time right now to go into this. You have a tour to take and I have to get ready to fly out for Europe. But I can tell you this and you can take it for what it's worth: There are events that *must* happen, and not all of them have been discussed in the current works on the subject. Actually, what it all comes down to when you're looking at the events is a gigantic gathering of Israel in preparation for the Second Coming. Remember what Moses said 'about a sweeping of the earth as with a flood'—speaking of our day—and for what purpose?" Samuel quickly answered his own question. "'To gather out God's elect from the four quarters of the earth.' What a program this is! Of course there will be upheaval, destruction, hardship, removal of peoples from the earth, but when you really analyze the events of the Second Coming, it comes down to a giant gathering and a dispensing of power and great righteousness like the world has only experienced once or twice. It really is a gathering of the elect like nothing ever before. Catch that vision of the leading events and you have the core of the Second Coming." Samuel let his breath out slowly. "It is so interesting. I stumbled upon something that absolutely must take place in the chain of events."

"Interesting. I'm fascinated, so tell me more."

"I will when we have time. I'll say this, though: Something so astounding has to happen before we even begin constructing the New Jerusalem, which has to be started before Christ comes in the clouds of heaven to usher in the thousand years of peace, that we'll all be astounded. Sid, I'm absolutely amazed that no one—I mean NOBODY—has mentioned it in any lecture, writings, or declarations; no, not any of the books on the subject have mentioned it. It is a fundamental and monumental event that must take place in the marvelous events leading up to the Second Coming. Yet, it is so clear to me now, I don't know how I ever missed it.

"Do you know that we lack the ability to even begin to receive the Savior at his Second Coming in our present state of mind? The gospel as we preach it right now offers the saints individual salvation, and only that. There is far more that is missing. It is something so huge, so marvelous for us as a people, that it has to first take place before there is a stone laid to build the New Jerusalem. You do know that the New Jerusalem—Phase One—has to be completed with the temple in place in Jackson County before Christ will come with the power of heaven? You'll be surprised when I tell you what this power of heaven is. Sid, I tell you, it is astounding and so vital. I came across it after literally years of study, contemplation, and prayer. Really, I did."

"What is this power of heaven?"

Samuel remained silent a moment.

"Don't leave me hanging."

"Yeah, I'll leave you hanging. I've given you a hint. So if you are really interested, you'll come to see me when we get home."

"Come on, that isn't fair. I'm interested in knowing right now."

"I know you are, but you'll just have to come to see me to get the answer. That's fair. If you are really interested, you'll come. Okay?"

\* \* \*

"The Paris Clinique." That was the phrase Katherine Moore used to describe to her lady friends in the Bay Area her favorite spot in Paris. Dr. Fournier's medical clinic off Rue Beaumont in the heart of Paris' fashion district took up one entire floor in the turn-of-the-century, four-story building. Katherine was a regular at this world-renowned cosmetic surgery center. She regularly made the flight from San Francisco to Paris for her "touch-ups." At the moment her body clock was so far off from the transatlantic flight two days earlier that the fact she had arrived at the clinic two hours ago, just after 7:00 in the morning, made little difference. Dr. Fournier had asked that she take another of the several sessions before he injected the Botox. She had begun the minor procedure of endermologies in San Francisco and had taken the final two under Fournier's supervision here in Paris.

She had done as he requested and was now back in his surgical unit following the sucking-and-rolling endermologies, a noninvasive procedure, at the hands of a highly skilled female therapist. She knew that the procedure was effective in reshaping the slight cellulite that crept into her slim hips. Though Katherine visited two plastics in an office near her penthouse in San Francisco, she reserved the new, the unique, the latest innovations in the art of reshaping one's body and face for this very special Dr. Fournier who sat perched on the corner of a long, white, rolling table in the center of his surgical room. There were mirrors on the ceiling and along two walls opposite one another in floor-to-ceiling sheets of glass. Dr. Fournier liked to point out to his patients, when he examined their final results, that life was like the mirrors facing each other. "You look into either one and see endless reflections. Beauty is like that. It is endless and eternal." Analyzed, his statements may have made little sense, but for Katherine this small, rather effeminate doctor had the touch and stretched his talents to achieve for Katherine the ultimate in enduring beauty. She knew that he was extremely careful to make realistic face improvements that were subtle but pronounced; the flattering looks that he re-created on her were for the long haul. She also knew that he was surgeon to some of the most famous and tautest faces in Hollywood. Yet, somehow he always took the time to give her special treatment. It perhaps had little to do with her ability to pay and more to do with her easy manner and simple charm.

Each time Katherine visited his clinic, the French doctor seemed compelled to take an extra few minutes to enjoy her company. This was Katherine, always a lady of charm who could attract friends. In her, charm was a primary feature that had attracted Samuel and other men before him. Fournier had the manner and skills that pleased her. This morning he had injected tiny amounts of Botox along the corners of the eyes and above the lips where small lines were forming—they would be gone by tomorrow. Months before, she had undergone laser resurfacing. However, Botox offered immediate results for the fine lines that had begun resurfacing along her cheeks.

"You know, for a lady in her sixties you look remarkably well preserved," Dr. Fournier complimented. His English sounded smooth and natural, with the hints of French that mellowed out the harsh consonants of English. "Part of your extended beauty is surgical; however, more importantly, the genes you were born with have combined, offering you a remarkable beauty that many envy. I think there are many women I see who would love to trade places with you, my dear," the doctor observed. Dr. Fournier's accent reminded Katherine of the once-famous French actor Charles Boyer. At the moment he arose, reached out to Katherine's face, and touched the smooth, creamy-white skin about her high cheek bones, examining the vanished lines, amazed at the freshness of her face. He knew that the world was kind to such beauty, that it smiled on those who, like this woman, were graceful in face and figure at any age.

The day before, Katherine had arrived at the clinic to get her touch-up shots of wrinkle-erasing Botox and two sessions in endermologies. With booster shots, she hadn't been able to scowl in the past two years. The numbed muscles along her brow had stopped trying. "I love being paralyzed in my forehead," Katherine raved. "I feel like with your help I look younger now at 65 and more youthful than I did at 50."

"I assure you that you do." Dr. Fournier tilted his head, studying Katherine's brow with a pensive look and said, "I'm certain you are right." He then moved his long, thin fingers to the center of her brow and pressed areas where wrinkles would have been deep grooves without his artistic, medical talents. He knew as a once-budding artist that there was symmetry to her face, so important among world-class beauties. He also knew well the art of correcting uneven results in surgeries that he may not have performed. Katherine had come to him over fifteen years before with some uneven surgery that an American cosmetic surgeon had botched. Fournier had done miracles with the face. She was among his most prized patients. Casually commenting, he mused, "You know, my mother insisted I take up painting and pencil drawing as a small child. I've always been grateful that she insisted on art first."

"I understand and I appreciate your mother's philosophy of beauty. My body has benefitted from her insistence." Katherine smiled. She turned from the mirrors to look into Fournier's long, handsome face; then she stretched out her hand to shake his. She wanted to get to a phone and call Samuel in Jerusalem, and preferred making the call from her hotel room rather than in the clinic— greater privacy. This was all the time she cared to spend with Fournier, though she enjoyed her moments chatting with him. Nevertheless, while still in Paris, she had people to see and places yet to go. "Thank you, Doctor. You've been most kind and, as usual, very creative."

# Chapter 2

The chilled morning air fell coldly on the face of the cliff east of Gateway in Wyoming, and the frosty mist cast an eerie glow on the compound buildings below. The muffled voices of the security personnel momentarily broke the silence of the Wyoming morning as the guard changed. Illuminated by the hazy sun that sent shafted rays of light along the base of the perimeter fence, the shadows of the shifting guards projected silhouettes that rose phantom-like on the glass walls of the spectacular Gateway Tower, a near replica of the Crystal Cathedral in Garden Grove, California.

Deep within the mountain behind the cliff, hidden within an enormous inner cavern, the prefab buildings of the indoctrination center lay in silence. Orange night lights along the walls of the cavern dimly illuminated the three military vehicles parked in formation toward the back. Behind them were the vaulted security doors protecting the communications chamber with its ultra-high-tech computers. Off to the side, accessible through a tunnel, was a smaller cavern with the grow rooms, their plants always warm and glowing. And beyond was an artificial pond surrounded by exotic plants and flowers. The air was filled with an almost intoxicating fragrance, totally alien to the Wyoming November.

This secret complex was the nerve center of the Grand Oracle's planned City of God. The pompous Oracle would welcome God upon his great return. The city would be waiting. But more than that, a people, a perfect people, would also be here to receive him. Of course the Oracle functioned on his five-year program, having calculated the time he had remaining to complete his complex plan to be on hand when the great millennial era arrived. Insane perhaps, yet so sinister and clever. There were those among his followers who truly believed he could pull it off. So far he had done what he had set out to do; with his inherited wealth he did in fact create a city worthy of note. City? Perhaps not that large, but the plans and the possibilities were there. Time was on his side by his inspired insight into the future. From this virgin spot of beautiful earth, surrounded by mountains, clear streams and pure air, he intended to reach out to the world with waves of light. His studies had convinced him that these waves could be used to control and direct the minds of all humankind. Crazy? Yes. But he was determined to see it through.

\* \* \*

Brenda Thorn was breathing uneasily, almost panting in her sleep. The outside beauty of Jackson Hole she never saw. It was dark and confining where they had locked her in. The cavern glow crept through the narrow window of her room in one of the prefab buildings and turned her pillow a pale yellow-orange. Alone and vulnerable, she lay face up with her arms extended above her head. She jerked her head nervously from side to side, emitting faint intermittent sobs and sighs. A strand of her glowing dark hair passed across her moist lips. She spit at it blowing to the side of her cheek.

It had been three weeks since she had consented to the Oracle Josiah's training, three weeks since she had seen the light of day. For Brenda it was in a twilight world, halfway between her old life of family comforts and now a strange, new life of spiritual renaissance.

Maybe.

It had sounded so exciting, had been so tempting to Brenda, who had considered herself a twenty-year-old truth seeker. But life in the Oracle's compound had not met her expectations. True, her days had been filled with intense mental stimulation, but her troubled sleep betrayed the battle raging within her soul. In her right hand she clutched a small photograph. It was forbidden. Many things were forbidden these past few weeks of confinement. To even think of family and friends was sinful.

A shadowy figure slipped quietly along the hallway of the prefab building and stopped before the doorway to Brenda's room. A hand reached for the doorknob and turned it ever so slowly. The door squeaked slightly on its hinges as it was pushed open. Brenda froze in her twilight sleep. The figure entered and walked to the foot of her bed. Two hands reached out and gently grasped Brenda's feet through the bed coverings and massaged them tenderly.

"What?" stammered Brenda as she suddenly awoke. "Who . . . ? Mother Martha, is that you?"

"Relax, Rachel," said the voice, using the name that had been assigned to Brenda in the compound. "It's me, Mother Martha. I heard you making noises in your sleep and I came. I'm here now. Let your mind be at peace. Think sweet thoughts of beautiful heavenly images. Visualize."

Heavenly images she could not muster. The practical side of her brain asked, "What time is it?" as she came to wakeful consciousness.

"Time is of no matter, not to us here," replied Mother Martha. "Relax. There is so much to learn in the classes tomorrow." The soothing voice shifted to a steady business-like tone. "But let's talk since you are wide awake." She reached over and turned on the lamp near Brenda's bed, revealing her own oval face, a narrow nose, very young-looking eyes surrounded by crow's feet earned in the sun-drenched regions of South America.

Brenda flinched in response to the sudden light shining in her blue eyes that she quickly covered with the back of her hand. Mother Martha had thought since first gazing at Brenda three weeks ago that her face was the embodiment of innocence. Mother Martha's own expression continued to be a study in tenderness as she looked down at Brenda, whose other arm was outstretched above her head. In contrast, Mother Martha's weathered face bore the marks of a harsh life, but her eyes glowed with feigned compassion. The two did not speak for a moment. Brenda removed her hand from her eyes and locked onto those of Mother Martha. Brenda slowly maneuvered the photograph with her thumb in her fisted hand above her head so it was out of sight. She clutched it tightly, hoping it was hidden inside her fist.

"Look at this portrait on your wall, Rachel," Mother Martha said in a kindly voice, pointing to the image of the Grand Oracle peering out at the viewer with deeply set black eyes. It was the sort of frontal shot of him that allowed the eyes to stare out at the viewer. "He will guide you in your sleep and in your waking hours. You need not fear."

"I'm not afraid, Mother Martha. It's just that I have not been outdoors for so long. Tomorrow I want to go out for a walk. You promised me. I need sunlight."

"Not tomorrow, child. Besides, you have the island to play on." She referred to the underground spa the Oracle had gone to great lengths to construct. "Tomorrow the Grand Oracle has scheduled a news conference with many visiting journalists. We must remain out of sight. The world is not yet ready to know all, and especially to learn of you. You are too special."

"But you promised I would be allowed to go outside." Brenda's voice nearly cracked with emotion. She added, "Do my parents know where I am? Have they called?"

"Your parents don't need to know where you are. It is not important for them to know. They are of the world. Remember, you are an adult and you have agreed to be here. Don't talk about family and friends. They no longer matter. You must get this firmly in your mind, my dear. Everything that matters is here, right here."

Brenda shifted her position nervously, lowering her arm to her side tightly concealing the photo, hoping she was not mutilating it in her grip.

Mother Martha saw the edge that protruded between the thumb and index finger. She shouted, "What are you holding there?"

"Nothing."

"Let me see it!" The witchy voice dominated.

"I have nothing to show you, Mother Martha."

"Child, let me see it!" She grabbed Brenda's clenched right fist with one hand and pried open the fingers with the other, one by one.

"No!" cried Brenda, almost frantically. "It is nothing!"

"Let me see that!" shouted Martha. She wrested the photograph from Brenda's hand and looked at it closely. The feigned compassion that had been so sugar sweet had shifted instantly to anger. "Your family! You still have a photograph of your family! I thought you had given me every possession you brought with you. You deceived me. This is unspeakable wickedness."

Brenda recoiled in horror as the witch maintained the iron grip on her wrist. "You're hurting me!"

"You know what I have taught you about family! You know the rules: No images of your family!" Releasing her grip on Brenda, the woman slowly and deliberately tore the photograph to shreds, scattering the remnants at random upon the blanket. Then she pointed to the portrait of the Grand Oracle on the wall. "That is your family! That is your father! That is your mother! That is your brother! That is your life! Can you not finally understand what I'm talking about?"

Brenda nodded quickly and nervously, her eyes wide and afraid.

"You know the penalty for retaining an image of your family, don't you?"

Brenda shrank positioning the back of her head against the wall, her brow furrowed, her eyes pinched shut, dreading the blow.

Mother Martha slapped her with the force of a Victorian nanny.

Brenda's scream echoed down the hall to the security desk and beyond. It sounded like some soul thrust down to hell.

* * *

Anney Thorn sat bolt upright in bed in her spacious home in the river bottoms of Provo. She had spent a troubled night. The alarm had not gone off yet; it was still too early in the morning. Her gasp penetrated the silence of the bedroom and jolted her husband, Stephen, out of a deep sleep. They had slept little through the night. Three different times the phone rang. Each time there was heavy breathing, but no voice could be heard. What kind of insensitivity must someone possess to pull such a trick in the middle of the night, especially with Brenda at who knows where?

"Anney, what's happening? What's wrong?" exclaimed Stephen, now fully awake.

She turned toward the faint, gray light from a night light in the bathroom. "I had a dream . . . about Brenda," she responded, still panting with frenzy. Stephen gathered Anney into his arms, his heart aching with compassion and concern that matched her own. The red digital numbers glowing on the night stand read 4:20 A.M.

"What was it about, honey?"

"I don't know . . . a nightmare, images, a darkness, Brenda in pain. Stephen, I'm so frightened. You don't know. I'm scared to death for Brenda."

Stephen continued to hold Anney closely and stroke her tousled blond hair. "I am afraid, too, Anney. But we don't really know where she is at this moment. For all we know she is sleeping peacefully in a warm bed."

"What are we going to do? There has to be some kind of a solution. There has to be."

She managed a faint hope in her voice. "My faith is not always as strong as it should be. But I do believe Heavenly Father will watch over our family, our Todd and Brenda. I do have faith. Really I do, Stephen. It's just that this is so hard, so terribly hard to endure."

"I love you, Anney," Stephen whispered soothingly. He kissed a salty tear from her cheek and tenderly drew her close.

"I love you too." She put her soft hand to his cheek and gently rubbed the short whiskers.

They settled back together on the pillows. He held her in his arms for a long while, until her breathing became slow and regular, then he pulled back his arm when he felt certain she was finally asleep.

Stephen closed his eyes and thought about a better future, about a society where such anxieties were a thing of the past, a society where families were together, a society of truth and light, a society of the City of Zion. For days now he had been working on the concept of the New Jerusalem and it tended to shadow his thoughts. How he longed for such peace and love that he was certain would prevail in the Holy City. Then he, too, finally drifted off to sleep.

* * *

Mother Martha had left the scattered, shredded pieces of the photograph strewn across the navy blue blanket. Brenda snatched up every tiny piece and laid them out like a puzzle on the table next to her bedstand. Mother Martha had turned off the lamp before leaving, but Brenda risked detection by security and had switched the lamp back on. She spent the next half hour piecing together the photo, wishing she had a sheet of paper and glue. She couldn't leave them out, so she gathered them up again after studying each person in the picture and stuffed the pieces deep inside her pillow case.

As they often did in fits of loneliness, Brenda's confused thoughts turned to Max and her family. The sting from Mother Martha's slap had subsided, but Brenda could not sleep. Troubled in mind, she had not been able to shake her desperate regret that she had blown it with Max. Had she been more insistent, more compelling, more loving, kinder, whatever it may have required, would she have been able to persuade him to marry her? No! Brenda knew there was a greater commitment in Max's life than their romance and possible marriage. He wanted to serve his God on a mission.

Little had she known how susceptible she had been to the small group who gathered that night in a student apartment and listened to a Gateway representative expound the Oracle's great hope for a brighter world. She thought something as exciting as the "Gateway experience" might offer an escape from her depression while getting over Max. It never entered her mind she was so susceptible to some sort of instant release from her very real world of school and a failed romance. Was she ready!

Yes, yes, yes. She needed a complete change in her life. The Oracle's representative had opened the door to a new opportunity, and Brenda had rushed in. Not only that, but by leaving college and going to Jackson Hole after writing the briefest of notes to her parents, she was trying to send a message. They had done much the same thing when they left the family religion and joined the Mormons, not to mention actually moving to the Mormon strong-hold, Utah. What thought had they taken of her reaction to their new-found belief? Zero. Zilch. Well, turn about was fair play . . . or was it?

Now, with real fear in her heart, Brenda reevaluated her course of action. What on earth had she done by consenting to join? What had she really committed herself to? How was she to get out of this pit and get back her life? She knew her parents would welcome her back. That was not the issue. Not right now. For several days now she sensed something was happening to her reasoning powers. Something had a grip on her thoughts and feelings. Unknown to her, life at Gateway—aided by drugs—was taking its toll on her mind, her resistance. She couldn't think straight. How was she ever going to escape back to her old world? Humdrum as it had seemed, it was a world she understood and now longed to have. It had never looked so good. How would she ever be the same again?

"Help!" she shouted to the walls. Her voice weakened as she slipped in and out of oblivion. "God in heaven, help me. Please help me," she whispered.

It had only been a few short weeks since Brenda had made the decision to join the Gateway group. But it seemed like a lifetime. She had mentally committed to investigate Gateway out of anger and frustration . . . right after the last time she spoke with Max, her boyfriend in Provo. She had felt such despondency the day she dialed his apartment. Brenda was grateful her younger brother, Todd, who roomed with Max, was still in class. Max had answered the call. Again and again she replayed the conversation in her mind:

"Hi."

"Oh, hi, Brenda. What's happening?"

The voice, the charm, the openness. These were the things Brenda loved about Max. She felt maybe this time they could talk . . . really talk. She hadn't spoken with him in nearly a week. He apologized for not calling her, explaining that time had gotten away from him, that college was a heavy scene for someone who had never graduated from high school.

"I understand," she had laughed. "I've been hitting the books too. But . . . I just thought since it's Friday and I'm missing you . . . that I would give you a call."

"Yeah, sure. I have a ton of stuff to get done for school, but I have time for you, Brenda."

Brenda misread his response, her spirits soaring. It sounded like he wanted to talk.

But she soon realized she was carrying the conversation. His comments were generally "yesses" and "noes." The more she talked, the more she was convinced he was not that glad to be on the phone with her. Girls have intuition. She prided herself on her ability to discern a phony attitude. All the time they spent together last summer gave her insights into traits that even he didn't know he had. One was his inability to fake sincerity.

Brenda finally came to the point. She knew she shouldn't force the issue, but she couldn't stop herself. It was like stepping off a cliff with her eyes wide open. A strange sensation—as if she could hear the very words she was about to say and his response.

"Max . . . ah . . . I have to ask. This thing we had going. . . . Is it over? Don't be afraid you'll hurt me. I need to know. I need a life too. So I'm asking you, how do you really feel about me?" Holding her breath, she sensed her question had come at him so suddenly, so completely off the wall, that he had to take a moment to phrase what she intuitively knew he would say. The pause lasted too long to be anything but negative. "Well?" she asked at length.

"Brenda, Brenda, why does it have to be a do-or-die thing? Why can't we be close friends and see where this thing goes after my mission?"

"No! No! No!" Brenda knew she was shouting, but failed to control her surging emotions. She could hear the fury in her voice; her head seemed ready to explode. "No, Max." Her voice had dropped to a whisper. "I can't just love you like a sister. It's over."

Max was too stunned at her outburst to reply. Before he could form an answer, she continued, this time in a harsh, bitter tone.

"You don't have to worry about me calling you anymore. I'm out of the scene. You . . . the whole bunch of you can take your holy attitudes and missions, . . . your fake brotherly kindness, and leave me out. That's it!" She slammed the phone down hard on its cradle and slowly lowered herself onto the couch, letting her head fall back in disbelief. She stared at the ceiling in her small, dorm-like apartment, alone, desperate to undo what she had done. The keen pain that shot through her body, beginning in her mind and coming to rest deep in her heart, felt like it must feel to be shot, to be electrocuted, to be stabbed. Pain is pain. In fact, at that very moment she would have preferred a gunshot wound. It would have been merely physical. This pain disturbed her thought pattern, it upset her power of reasoning, it drove her nearly mad with fear. If only Max would call back, but he didn't.

What followed must have been fate. How else would the Gateway people have known to include her with the select group of kids who were considering a lifestyle change? The following Saturday she  accepted their invitation to attend a meeting, where only four other students were present. There a man smoothly explained man's greatest hopes and joys about life and death and how a wise Oracle had constructed for his God a magnificent, tiny city whose gates were open to the few, the very few. . . .

Brenda had been swept up with the group. She had committed to enter the order, especially after the representative had shown a video of the Oracle and Gateway surrounded by mountains and streams, the Grand Tetons in the background, the wonderful skies and happy young members. Some were so good looking in the photos. On screen the Oracle himself had been powerful, mesmerizing.

Brenda left school and apartment without telling her roommate. She took her small overnight suitcase and left the apartment while her roommate was gone. She was told she needed none of her clothing, nor her stereo system, her books—nothing. All would be provided for her new life.

# Chapter 3

"Samuel! Samuel!" Katherine's light, melodious voice drifted across the lobby of the Estil Hotel in Paris where she was a guest. Immediately Samuel smiled, though his back was to her. The voice, oh the charm in that voice!

Samuel turned about slowly, put both hands on his hips, and smiled with that knowing grin on his face, shaking his head. She suddenly swept across the marble floor to greet him. He teased, "You certainly fit the environment of this city."

She came up to him with her arms wide. They embraced a moment. At the front desk, across the lobby, Brad observed the scene when he heard Katherine exclaim his grandfather's name. He felt uncertain about this woman—this lady in his grandfather's life. Her elegance and seeming charm weren't lost on Brad. She had an air of finely tuned charm and good looks that even he, at 23, could detect. Maybe there was too much charm there. He nevertheless saw that his grandfather was smitten by her, and in some crazy way that pleased him. Still, he was protective of his grandfather's emotions and hoped this was not going to create problems for this man he loved dearly.

"How is the handsomest man in the room doing, anyway?" Katherine said with sincere feeling as she looked into Samuel's creased, masculine face, touched his cheek with her right hand adorned with a large diamond on the ring finger, and then patted his face.

"I think there are those who dispute that I'm all that good looking," Samuel corrected as he tilted his head to one side toward the front desk where Brad had turned to face the clerk as he completed signing in. "My grandson Brad is over there. I want you to meet him."

"Oh, Samuel, I'd love to meet him."

"You'll meet them all. They'll all be at my place in Boise during Thanksgiving."

"I can hardly wait. I was glad you were traveling with your grandson. Israel is a time bomb waiting to go off. I don't like to think of you off in Israel alone."

"Don't worry, sweetheart. Everywhere I go lately I have friends to meet me and dine me and, you know, . . . really lay out the red carpet. But it has been great to be with Brad." Samuel tugged at Katherine's elbow in an effort to move her toward the front desk.

"My word, Samuel, from here he looks like he's a foot taller than you."

"Yeah, I think he is, or maybe eight inches taller. It comes from his mother's side—Hey, I thought we'd have dinner tonight. You name it and we'll go. I know you know your way around this town. Maybe we could even take in the opera if we can get tickets. What do you say? I hope you don't mind Brad tagging along. He's never been to Paris. He needs someone like you to show off the city."

"Of course I don't mind. I'd love to go anywhere with you. Besides, we'll have plenty of time to be alone in the next few weeks. I'm not going back to my place in San Francisco. Anney and Stephen have invited me to spend a few weeks at their place. Anney wants me to help her unpack. Oh joy."

* * *

Samuel had lingered at the door studying Katherine's face. Their evening together at the Ibarro restaurant and the stroll back to the hotel, elegantly dressed and in love, was one of those evenings when the whole world seemed to remain at a distance to allow the two to enjoy each other. Brad, after all, had not wanted to leave his room. He decided to do a cursory review of his taped scenes on his hand-held video to make notes for the cutting room when he returned to UCLA. He ordered in dinner.

Samuel leaned one arm against the wall next to the door to Katherine's room. He stood with only a couple of inches separating his lips from hers. Close, of course, Katherine's face was mature and the fine lines were gone, leaving her face with its natural tenderness and glow. The lips were full and inviting. He loved her smile, her wit, her complete self. He had fallen in love with her the first night they sat across from each other at that small table on board her ship. Love had come so naturally, so spontaneously. Now, three months later, the lure of her person and the charm of her soft voice sent Samuel, a widower, longing to be with this woman forever. He had not rushed into a relationship. For one thing, Katherine was not a member of the Church. This fact alone had caused a slight tapping on the brakes in their relationship, he knew, and he wondered if she had sensed it. Perhaps not.

It had been more than two years since Margaret's death. He had been certain he could never love another woman as he had loved her. Tonight he knew that was sheer nonsense. Why had he ever thought he couldn't love again? This dream before him reached up and tenderly put her lips to his. It sent a surge of passion through Samuel that he knew he had to guard against. Her touch alone had an electric feel to it.

"I love you, Samuel," she said with sincere joy in her tone of voice.

Samuel pulled her close and let his hand caress her neck as they stood embraced, "I love you, too. Oh, I just want us to be together always. Yet . . . "

She drew back. "What?"

"Nothing. I don't want to spoil the moment."

"Nor do I."

They stood close in the ornate hallway of the hotel for as long as Samuel felt his passions could endure. He released his grip on her shoulder and neck, leaned back, and she in turn let go of his arm and hand. She knew Samuel would not cross over the line he had drawn for his high sense of morality. She accepted this fact in their relationship and said, "Thanks for coming this evening to be with me."

"I had no choice. My heart brought me right to your arms. . . . But, I think I had better say goodnight. You are so—I'll say goodnight."

The face so porcelain-like, the lips a perfect fullness. The makeup was never too thick; the bright silver hair always in place, short but still full bodied. Samuel knew he could stand right there at the door to her room and gaze on her for an hour, even more. "Katherine, you are the loveliest thing I have seen on this entire trip. What can I say?"

"I feel the same about you and where we are. This is one of my favorite cities in the whole world." She lifted her hand and let it slip around Samuel's neck; then she pulled his head closer to give him a second kiss. "I know people will talk about you and me together here in Paris, but who has to know? We are old enough to be sensible. I love you, Samuel. Really, I do."

\* \* \*

It was one of those south-side walk-ups that flourished during the 1920s and '30s. The only light in the building cast a faint glow from Devin Kirk's office/bedroom tenement to the wet street below. Kirk was in and, as usual, hunched over his computer. He preferred doing his dirty deeds throughout the night. Out of bed in the late afternoon, he dressed and as usual lounged at a corner bar two blocks from his walk-up apartment. Never married, always hiding, Kirk possessed a skill that made him enough cash—always cash—to get by. His talent in life was forgery, in his case handwriting. He could clone the hand of most anyone in English, provided he was given enough original script from the writer whose hand he forged. He had learned as a kid in the Bronx from bond forgers how to style and curve the written letters of others. He had made a meager living at the skill for so long that he wasn't at all certain just what his own original handwriting resembled. He had one other talent that came with the pathetic package he called his creative, darkened mind: He could whip out a believable story line, especially in brief letters, that sounded like the person he was deceivingly composing for.

Tonight he had to compose and forge handwriting for only eight of the "students" at Gateway, though he didn't know that was the name of the location where his subjects were housed. In fact, he didn't know about the Oracle. He worked strictly with a guy who divulged nothing but names and addresses and reams of pages of student notes and letters that students thought they were writing home. He had been doing this for over two years and now had a fair idea that some of the kids for whom he forged letters were not happy to be in the compound out West.

This late hour's load of letters to be written was light, considering he wrote in the young person's writing style and manner of expression over a hundred letters a week. He mailed them from his local mail drop in a variety of locations in Chicago to confuse any possible search to a lady in St. Louis who posted them from the central post office in her city to parents all over the country, but mostly on the West Coast.

Kirk had placed his black lamp to shine from the edge of his computer table onto several handwritten notes from one Brenda Thorn. A cute little gal, Kirk noted from her University of California at Redlands student ID photo that smiled out at him from the corner of some class notes that were laid out as guides for imitation. They were class notes Brenda had handwritten while she was still enrolled at school a few months earlier.

He knew next to nothing about the man he worked for. All he knew was that each week he received the code word "Bandit" on his e-mail and the initials in reverse of those students who were sending mail to their parents. This gal's reversed initials were TB, meaning Brenda Thorn. In all of Chicago, only Kirk knew that TB were the reversed initials of a young girl somewhere in the West, locked in some compound and not allowed to write her own parents. Kirk did that for her, and he would make her sound so happy to be with a secluded group of kids in some fantasy compound that didn't exist. This was what Kirk did best, and he got by on the money he received to make his meager ends meet.

Kirk knew he was composing these letters for a guy he had known in New York, one Hap Kobler, a man who got busted a couple of times for violation of immigrant labor exploitation. Kirk was no dummy. He suspected Hap had committed worse crimes than simply taking fifty percent of the wages his Central American immigrants earned on the streets of New York. Well, it was time to get at it.

In one swig, Kirk finished off his lukewarm mug of coffee, pulled up a blank screen, and began from Word. He liked Word; it had a spelling and grammar checker that underlined his mistakes as he wrote out the letters on the screen. At times Kirk deliberately misspelled certain words that certain young people misspelled in their own writings. If nothing else, Kirk had learned as an apprentice to be consistent.

Kirk would type out the brief letter, print it, reread the hard copy, then move across his cluttered room to a cheap composition table he used as a handwriting desk. Hand composition was the most difficult part of his trade in deception. He would handwrite each letter he created. At times he had to write a second time. In this one area of his miserable life he was a perfectionist. He addressed the envelope and stuffed it in the packet he mailed out every three days to St. Louis.

For some reason, Kirk's fake letters home to mommy and daddy weren't flowing as usual. Maybe it was the gal staring up at him from her photo on the sheet. Kirk turned over the plastic-encased picture. Still, he couldn't get the swing of it. He made two wrong S's as he wrote with blue ink from a Bic. He began a second time with the usual Brenda "Hi Mom & Dad . . . " He was feeling better about the flow as he copied from his computer print-out letter. It was a short letter. Some were. He had told the parents about the wonders of living in a communal group in the woods and how inspiring everyone was, et cetera, et cetera.

* * *

The 727 banked and headed west. It continued to climb out of Kennedy where Samuel, Brad, and Katherine had cleared customs on their way to Kansas City. The plane leveled off at 34,000 feet, far above the storm that blanketed all of the eastern seaboard. Earlier, they had slept most of the trip from Paris to New York. The last night in Paris, then up at 3:00 in the morning, they had caught the earliest flight to New York. The wide seats of first class had their advantages. The food had not been Parisian, only fair. Katherine had taken her pill the moment the 747 leveled off over France, and with a few bites of breakfast she had dozed off. Samuel just naturally slept well anytime he felt like he needed the rest. Brad listened on the headphones across the aisle from them until he grew weary and dozed off as well.

They had cleared customs early morning (New York time) and were again in flight by midmorning. to spend the day in the Missouri countryside. Katherine had no idea of what to expect in some remote meadow in the middle of Missouri. She really didn't care. She was with Samuel and that was really all that mattered at the moment. He had warned her before inviting her to come along. "You may prefer to go directly home to San Francisco, dear. Brad and I have to stop off and get some footage of a location in Missouri, a place that has real significance to the Mormons." During their wait at Kennedy, she had actually taken a room at the Sheraton Airport Hotel for half an hour and took a shower, did her makeup, and had rejoined Samuel and Brad at the gate, ready for the day.

During this leg of the flight home, Katherine had been on the phone to Anney. The phone was the sort the airline conveniently provided on the back of the seat in front of her. After Anney had explained the lack of information on Brenda and her deep concerns, and Katherine had offered her shoulder for ten more minutes, Anney purposely shifted the conversation away from the Brenda issue back to Katherine's stay in Paris. Katherine chatted on about her Paris doctor and the fact that she had also closed the deal on the *Free Eagle*. Then she suddenly stopped and turned to Samuel, who was jotting down notes about his upcoming presentation tomorrow night to the authors and scholars who might tear him into tiny pieces when he presented some of his findings, and said, "Here, Samuel. Stephen wants a word with you." Katherine handed over the receiver to Samuel who leaned sideways in his seat, took the phone from Katherine's hand, and spoke.

"Stephen, hi."

"Hi, Samuel. How was your trip?"

"Great. I'll tell you all about it when I get in. I just want you to know when you meet with those contractors that we have already scheduled to start digging the basement. I've had some experience with contractors. You have to be careful; they will promise you deadlines they can't meet. I wish I were going to be there. I was delayed in Paris and I'm very sorry I can't make the meeting."

"Sure, no problem. I'll do that," Stephen replied, his strong bass voice came over the satellite with clarity. It shouldn't have surprised Samuel that the phone system on an aircraft was little different than one on the ground. Still it intrigued him that he could stay in touch so easily these days. Almost too easily. Where does one go for total privacy?

"I wish you were here, too," Stephen lamented. "But I'll be with them in a little over an hour. I'm sure we could reschedule if you want me to."

"No. Just don't sign anything. Okay?"

Samuel leaned forward to replace the phone on the rear of the seat in front of Katherine. He tipped the phone in her direction. He nodded as if he were offering her a drink. "You want to talk some more?"

"No. Go ahead and hang it up. I just want to relax. It's been a long flight from Paris. Usually, I take the polar route from Paris to San Francisco. It seems shorter, especially if I take a pill my doctor prescribes."

"Well, don't take a pill on this two-hour flight, darling. You might not wake up."

Katherine edged her fingertips across the arm rest and gently rubbed the back of Samuel's hand in a caressing manner. "Have I told you lately that I love you?"

"Yeah, but I like the sound of it anytime."

\* \* \*

The Oracle sat alone, pondering, staring out the floor-to-ceiling windows that brought the illusion of having the outdoors inside. The enclosed atrium sparkled with falling snowflakes, covering whatever green flora remained from fall. Spots from each corner of the enclosed garden cast enough light into the massive chrome-and-brass office to reveal the Oracle staring out at the chilling night as he let images of glory sink into his brain. The most obvious physical features of the man up close were the steady eyes and extended forehead. At 60 he looked as he had at 40, only grayer and slightly thinner. Tall and erect, he commanded a powerful presence. Even alone in his office there was an aura of power and determination in his demeanor. It had always been that way. Coming from old money, there was within him a sense of privilege and influence.

The sound of chimes echoed around the room. The Oracle pulled himself from his silent thoughts and said in a quiet voice, "Come in." As he said the words, he released the electric lock that secured the office from any intruder. The lock was set to automatically lock from the inside whenever someone entered from the outer office where the Oracle's personal secretary usually sat. It was near sunrise. She had left the office over six hours ago. Reuben entered. He was head of security and a sometimes bodyguard of the Oracle. But not often. Reuben's job, as head of the security force, required an increasing amount of time to control the entire compound the Oracle had created. To hear Reuben tell it, he had a job that required time and a half to merely keep ahead of the pack, particularly with outside forces that were bent on disrupting the Oracle's sacred mission, a mission to prepare a house for the Lord to come to when the Millennium commenced. Reuben didn't buy such crap, but the money was good, living space excellent, and he enjoyed total control of most of what went on in the compound. This was heady stuff for him.

"I got your call. Something wrong?" Reuben asked as he crossed the room, lightly padding on the silky, soft, Chinese carpet with colors of wine that covered all but a foot of oak floor on each of the four sides of the room. This century-old piece had been in the Oracle's family for three generations. No one could set a price on such a work of art, or for that matter on the other rare pieces that adorned the otherwise ultramodern suite. The Oracle had been reared by one of America's most private, wealthy families whose lives were purposely kept within secure walls where no snoop ever got a glimpse of the opulent life the Oracle had grown up with.

The Oracle responded, "I wish to high heaven I had insisted we not have those curious, aggressive journalists visiting us today. I know, I gave the approval—don't remind me. We agreed it would be good PR. But I've had second thoughts, deep reservations about this whole open house concept. We don't need PR, not at this time. We are a power unto ourselves. Why should we open our gates to these people whose business it is to expose our most sacred charge?"

"It's too late for that, sir; they are coming in a few hours. I've got security in force, and I doubt there is any better security in the country than what we will have while those inquisitors are snooping around. I assure you, sir, they will see only what we have already determined they should see. You have my word on this."

* * *

Sheriff Horn Harmon, in his early fifties, was a burly man with deep wrinkles and leathery skin who looked as tough as the Grand Tetons to the north of his office. He grew up on the slopes of the Grand Tetons and got into law enforcement from being a MP in the military. Harmon had twenty-seven years of county law enforcement behind him, half of it behind this desk and the rest out on the streets and back roads of the still rather wild regions of Jackson Hole. The local dialect, which was slow and drawn out, came through loud and clear as he spoke into the phone with Jackson's police chief, Wally Reinholdt. Leaning back, Harmon sat behind his wide oak desk in his recently renovated office at the rear of the county building that occupied one whole city block.

The complex, comprising courthouse, jail, and law-enforcement offices, had been situated near the center of Jackson Hole for over seventy years. Parts of it showed their age, especially around the framed windows where old, once-white paint curled in the sharp autumn air.

Sheriff Harmon was telling the chief of police about the visit he had earlier in the day with a Mr. Massey who had flown in from the regional office of the Federal Bureau of Investigation in San Francisco to spend a few hours with him. There was a residue of resentment by the city police chief toward Harmon, who had been rather direct during President Clinton's visit when two of the chief's police officers refused to direct traffic under county authority. The friction abated, but slight resentment remained. Still, the two law enforcement officers had to remain cooperative. Each knew the other depended on a reciprocal arrangement to enforce the law. Overlap was inevitable.

"What did he want, Horn?"

"He wanted to acquaint himself with our law enforcement setup here in Jackson Hole because we have jurisdiction over that damn Gateway compound. This Massey fellow—he was all FBI—let me know he has twenty-three years with the Bureau."

"So? Who cares?"

"Yeah, well, I guess he's the West Coast's leading troubleshooter for self-styled prophets like that mental case out at the compound. . . . I guess he's a kind of expert on these guys that head up religious orders and defy the law if it gets in their way. It was this Massey fellow who handled that recent invasion of the neo-Nazi group in Carson Valley. You remember, that bunch down there in Nevada? I hope to hell we don't have that kind of situation out at Gateway."

There was a grunt on the other end from the city police chief.

"I know. It's not your jurisdiction, right? Anyway, Massey said he has information on that kook out there that makes the BATF in Washington nervous. They are asking me to personally look into Gateway without stirring up a hornet's nest. The FBI has a thick file on the Oracle. They claim he's a dead ringer for a megaproblem. All they want to do is keep the lid on the situation. I told him that there ain't a whole lot we can do to stop what they're doing out there to all those young people unless we get some complaints. That shooting over in Nevada, I understand, netted them that guy on federal firearms charges. They caught him with a ton of illegal weapons and the guy panicked. He wounded a couple of BATF agents during a shootout when they attempted to arrest him. I read about that in the paper. Anyway, I guess the guy who was caught with the goods was advised by his shiny-suited attorney to cop a plea. But he must have sung, because he said to the FBI that he had sold weapons to the folks out at Gateway. Automatics. Turns out this informant," Harmon went on, "who is still going to spend a fair amount of time in lockup, had sold our local resident, the Oracle, some modified weapons. The Oracle paid the informant to alter a bunch of legal semiautomatics to illegal, fully automatic machine guns. From what he told the boys in the FBI, the deal was made at a gun show where the informant was a gunsmith showing off his wares. They got cozy; the informant made a trip up here as a guest of the Oracle and saw the whole show. He says they were in a cave . . . at least, he thinks it was a cave. If it's true, we've got ourselves an explosion waiting to happen."

"I'm aware of that. I read about the arrest, too," the chief said, making no effort to disguise his indifference to the whole situation at the compound. "What do you mean, he thinks he was in a cave? I've heard there are caves out there, but I was never in one. I don't think they're very large."

"Well, the Oracle was cagey enough to blindfold the guy. He said the Oracle talked about his hefty stash of military hardware, but our informant actually saw nothing."

"Great. This leads nowhere. Hey, Horn, this is all very interesting, but I'm glad as hell that Gateway is in your jurisdiction and not mine."

"I may need your help if things get exciting out there. The guy in prison I'm certain did modify the weapons, and I'm sure the Oracle didn't flush them down the toilet. They're out there. We just have to get into the place and take a look around."

"I repeat, it's your jurisdiction. I'll help, but . . . "

"Just a damn minute here!" Harmon shouted. Through force of habit, he glanced around as he swore, though he was alone in his secure office. He had no patience with Reinholdt's lack of concern. "Listen, Wally, this Massey said the feds have reason to believe that somewhere around that compound he has stashed some assault vehicles with missile launchers on them. The informant said the Oracle was bragging about the military equipment he had and he mentioned assault vehicles specifically. Who knows what he's got out there?"

"But he saw nothing?" the chief responded.

"That's right. But they intend to get incriminating evidence by convincing someone inside the place to talk. Based on information they have from the snitch, they're sure the Oracle is capable of launching missiles. When this gunsmith they arrested started talkin', he spilled everything he knew."

"Sounds to me like he spilled more than he knew. Come on, Horn. Do you really think this Oracle fellow is that dangerous? He may be a kook, but he's not stupid from what I hear. They've never done anything, to my knowledge, for you to get too excited. They seem bent on peace and love—the old sixties idea of happiness. Don't go stirring up something that—"

"I just thought I'd call and let you know about my visit with this Massey follow."

"Well, I appreciate that."

"I don't know exactly what's happening, but I do know one other thing that got me stirred up."

"What?"

"Massey says the Bureau sees a pattern forming of college students who have disappeared from school, and the parents don't have the foggiest idea where their kids have gone, though all the parents say they get mail from their kids from somewhere in the Midwest, telling their folks everything is okay with them."

"Then why would Massey think this Oracle has them inside his compound?"

"Because one of the things this informant mentioned in passing was that all of the kids, boys and girls, he saw in the main hall before he was blindfolded were all about the same age, around their early twenties."

"So, does this Massey think that all the college kids who have disappeared are out there at Gateway?"

"He didn't say that. The guy is paid to suspect anything and anybody. He's just going for a long shot."

"That's a pretty long shot, Horn. Didn't he say the kids were writing their folks from the Midwest?"

"Yeah, but they've checked for return addresses, and none of the letters have a return address."

"Okay. It sounds like a crazy, mixed-up bunch of people is all stirred up. What do you want from me?"

"Massey wants information, but warned me to be cautious. That's why I'm calling you. Can you and your officers help us a little?"

"How?" Reinholdt asked warily.

"Massey wants to know who all's coming to town from Gateway and what they're doing. He's looking for anything unusual. And we have to do it without anyone noticing us. I want your help, chief. If any of those kids come to town—or, for that matter, anybody else from out there—we want to know it. We may even go so far as to pick one of 'em up."

"On what charge?"

"I'll get back to you on the charge. Anyhow, can you give me some time tomorrow? I'll come over to your office. I just want to fill you in on everything so we can coordinate our efforts."

"Sure, I'm with you," Wally said grudgingly. "But I sure as hell don't want to get my boys and girls involved in some standoff. I don't want a jurisdictional problem either, and you're asking me to step out on a limb. Personally, I'm not afraid of the so-called Oracle. I do think the guy is insane and needs to be put away. I'll help. But there are limits."

"Good. I need some cooperation, that's all."

"Sure. I understand where you're coming from."

\* \* \*

The midday sun felt warm in the sky this November day, though there were clouds forming in the west. It had the usual feel of a Midwestern autumn—crisp air, sparse leaves where there had been a profusion of color a month before; maples, elms, and other natural vegetation spread out before them. It was a seasonal image in the Midwest, in contrast to what Samuel had felt and seen in Jerusalem's dry, desert air several days before. In a few minutes the brooding clouds would block out the sun and roll through the valley. Samuel had rented a small Buick after he, Katherine, and Brad disembarked from their flight from New York. They had driven to this small valley, nearly a hundred miles from Independence, Missouri, to show her ADAM-ONDI-AHMAN. They walked from the board poster that displayed the name of the location to a nearby field. Samuel chatted with Katherine as they neared the center of the meadow. Brad lugged the camera while the grandfather toted the batteries and filming equipment.

Samuel mentioned, as the three moved though the field, how he had heard that members of the Church actually served gardening missions to keep up the site. Katherine found it intriguing that the Church took such an interest in this particular site, a site that Samuel had spent the last hour, while driving, explaining some of the Church history.

Sparsely leafed trees lined the path that led to the center location where Samuel pointed out where on the bluff an altar once stood, the sacred altar that Father Adam had constructed to worship the Lord. They halted their stroll in the center of the meadow where in warmer weather the grass grew tall and wild flowers bloomed. This mid-fall day the grass was changing from a deep green to a straw yellow. November had taken its toll on the otherwise inviting field. "I want you to begin filming as I walk around the mount, Brad. Okay? Then do a sweeping view of the whole valley."

Samuel had become something of an expert on the entire future of the Church in Missouri. "I don't say a whole lot about this to most people I talk to. The Church has always advised us to keep things simple and factual." Samuel glanced down. Pointing his finger at the yellow grass, he said, "It may have been about here that Adam built an altar and gathered his children about him. Yeah, I'd say about here." He crooked his neck to get a full view of Katherine, who was looking at him with a puzzled expression.

Katherine, in heather-tone jacket and stretch velvet pants, reached out to touch the elbow of Samuel's heavy wool-melton-blend jacket zipped to his chin. "You really believe we are standing on sacred ground, don't you?"

"I really do, sweetheart." Samuel spread his arms wide and turned a complete hundred and eighty degrees as he said, "It was here in this natural splendor that Adam gathered his children in a Grand Council. It was three years before he died that he counseled with, among others, Seth, Enos, Cainan, Mahalaleal, Jared, Enoch, and Methuselah."

"Methuselah? You mean the same person I've heard of all my life, the oldest man to ever live on earth—that Methuselah?"

"That's right. He lived a lot longer after the grand council. But at the time of the grand council all the great men of that time gathered here."

"What were they doing here?" Katherine was more impressed with Samuel's conviction that it actually happened on this spot than she was with who had been present. She felt as if she were standing with a man who was visionary, certain in everything he spoke. It truly amazed her that he was so convinced. It was ethereal and charming. It was this trait in Samuel that caught her imagination. To Katherine it didn't matter whether they were seated in first class on an international flight from Paris to New York, or here standing in a simple field in the heartland of America. She loved Samuel and realized it was his complete dedication to what he believed and how he seemed to speak as if he had been an eyewitness to some of the world's great events that set her heart swirling in affection toward him. If Samuel believed Adam stood right where they were standing, so be it. "What else happened here?"

"Well, for a starter, the Lord appeared. He came for the express purpose of blessing Adam and called him Michael, the prince, the archangel."

"Adam must have stood in good with the Lord once again to have had such a visit."

Samuel let a smile curl up on one side of his lip as he looked over at Katherine. "You don't really believe this, do you?"

"I believe in you, darling. If you are convinced the Lord came down and stood here"—Katherine made a quick side step as if she were clog dancing—"right here, does it make any difference whether I personally believe and accept your wonderful description of the events?"

"To me it makes a big difference. I want you to feel what I feel, know what I know, and thrill with the sensation of comprehending some of the most significant events in all history."

"Well, you have high hopes for a plain, little old lady who has not spent a lifetime delving into these things. Don't be disappointed, my love, if I come from a little different perspective; don't worry. We're together out in nature, and you're telling me things that are dear to your heart. What else matters?"

Samuel knew he had brought Katherine to this location as much to be with her as to tell of the glorious events that would one day transpire in this very valley. He knew better than to expect too much from her in these matters. Enjoy the moment, he told himself. Enjoy.

Samuel looked over at his grandson. He wondered what Brad thought of the way Katherine explained her reaction to this sacred location. Well, he would learn before long that Katherine was one who expressed her feelings, no matter where. "Brad, I think we're ready to start filming. Come in close and pick up the sound. If it is faint or soft, we'll dub at the studio. Do your best."

Brad stepped a few feet forward with the lens zooming in to frame Samuel's face only. He began filming.

\* \* \*

Burton threw up his large hand as if he were in a classroom. He wanted the Oracle's attention at this special luncheon for the visiting journalists who had been granted a rare opportunity to have an audience with Josiah, the self-styled, charismatic, religious leader whom Burton knew that everyone referred to as the Oracle. The Oracle had finished answering a female journalist from the *Seattle Express*. She sat five tables away from Burton, who was centered under the vaulted glass ceiling. She had asked how the Oracle raised funds to sustain the activity and why Gateway's religious compound was built at the base of the eastern cliffs of Jordan Creek, fifteen miles from Jackson in the Jackson Hole region. He had a ready answer: God told him where to built the compound.

The Oracle spoke, "God blessed my family with wealth. I have now inherited that wealth and with it I have built this residence for my God. As his chosen servant I have consecrated this magnificent edifice to the Second Coming." Burton felt, as he listened to the Oracle present the details of his project, that the self-appointed servant skimmed over the essential details of sustaining a compound that sported perhaps the most striking building in all of the region with its replication of the Crystal Cathedral look. The group sat at linen-covered tables with red-rose centerpieces flown in from the sunnier climes of California. In the main dining hall—which was usually occupied by the sixty or so young people who were members of the order—Burton sat with the other media folk who were guests for the day.

The Oracle was a tall, lean figure with penetrating eyes, possessed with an arrogant stance. He nodded and pointed his manicured index finger in Burton's direction. "Yes?"

Taking his cue without hesitation, Burton was on his feet, projecting his voice like Stephen A. Douglas debating Abraham Lincoln. "How many members are there in this order, and why are most of the young people here about the same age, which I'm guessing is somewhere around late teens to early twenties?" As he asked the question, Burton was increasingly aware that there was something almost mystical about the leader of this youthful group. He hoped to expose a crack in the man's facade.

The Oracle brushed back his almost-white hair with his hand, a reflex that allowed a pause before responding to the question. He was unaware of the little hand-hair movement, but he often unconsciously resorted to it. It was a minor gesture, but those closest to him on his staff noticed it, even though (naturally) none of them ever brought it to his attention. "We have currently . . . " He turned to his chief of security, the one they called Reuben, seated at the head table and asked for a precise count. Reuben declared with a sharp, gravelly, smoker's voice that there were sixty-four members in the compound.

"Thank you. There you have the count. As to age, no one in the compound is under the age of 20, according to our records."

Since he had the floor, Burton remained standing to toss out a question for his companion, Roy. A man in his mid-twenties, Roy lacked the assertiveness of Burton and let Burton ask the questions.

Burton had been a journalist for over six years and loved the arena of question/answer. The two men had come together on this journalistic tour for the day; Burton for a story, Roy for information on a man-made city of God.

Again Burton's voice boomed with the question, "Sir, we've noticed there don't seem to be sixty-four members present on the grounds or in this building. Where are the others?"

Again the Oracle's hand went to his hair, a smile frozen on his face. He didn't welcome these types of queries. The fact that Reuben had assured him it would be good PR to have the press in, answer a few simple questions, and let them look over the facilities, at least those areas they had predetermined would be okay for journalists to view, didn't relieve his disquietude. But he knew he had to respond to Burton's probe. In an icy voice he replied, "Over half of our members are in classes, assignments in the kitchen, and other locations. They are attending to their individual responsibilities. Surely you can understand that essential tasks have to be performed, that all things do not halt simply because we have guests on the premises."

Burton was not easily put off. He took one more shot at the Oracle. "Will we be allowed to see these young people at work or in their classroom setting?"

"No!" the Oracle quickly responded with irritation in his voice. Then catching himself, he softened his voice. "We have invited you to see our city we call Gateway. But it is a sacred space here on earth, and there are areas of this holy city that are not to be disturbed by outside influences. This is a near-monastic order. You understand, don't you? May I say that we only ask that you respect the sanctity of these hallowed grounds and be content with a tour of our facilities. Thank you."

The Oracle began to lower himself into his chair at the center of the head table. He had answered enough questions. Besides, the questions could last all afternoon if he didn't halt them soon. Another question was voiced. It was Morris

Turnbull of *The Oakland Herald*. He spoke without rising to his feet. Seated close to Burton, he blurted out his question before the Oracle could end the interview.

"Tell us, if you will, why you think God would be interested in occupying this piece of ground and buildings when he comes a second time. I thought he was to come to his sacred temple in Jerusalem."

All eyes turned to Turnbull, whose question had hit the core of an issue that was in their collective minds. How could a mere man think God would appear in his private dwelling spot located, of all places, in Wyoming . . . not in Israel or, for that matter, in some other more exalted location on earth?

Eyes then shifted to the Oracle, awaiting a response. The Oracle, too, remained seated as he responded. By sitting down, he had signaled a close to all queries. Yet this journalist, seated at what the Oracle was perceiving as a rebellious table, had the audacity to continue the interrogation. Indignantly, the Oracle began his response, "Throughout the Bible, God has selected an individual to lead the way. Though Gateway may appear to be somewhat ordinary . . . "

" . . . No, I don't think it is ordinary at all. It's pretty impressive," Turnbull interrupted. "It's obvious that megabucks have been spent on this building alone." His hands shot into the air, gesturing the magnificence of the building.

The Oracle nodded with little patience for the man who spoke with a tone of cynicism. "God has been known to appear in rather obscure places," the Oracle continued as if the Oakland newsman had not interrupted him. "I have it by sheer insight, that does not emanate from man, that God is pleased with this location and what we are doing here. He will appear one day. I want to welcome him and bestow that privilege on those who follow in my footsteps. I feel quite certain he will appear in my lifetime. No more questions, please. Enjoy your lunch."

# Chapter 4

Roy Carver, Dr. Polk's assistant since the first project in San Diego, turned his long, angular face about and looked in both directions as he walked with quick steps along the shiny hardwood floor of the wide hall. The visit to the compound at Jackson Hole was coming to a close. Regardless, he needed a rest room. He had first tried the lounge area of the glass-and-steel building, hoping to find the rest room. No luck. He simply couldn't find it. He had wandered in the direction of a wing of the building that led to the north end. A girl in a blue silk robe and gold-threaded slippers stepped silently in front of him as he started to enter the wing. She seemed to appear out of nowhere. "Sir, may I help you?" With an ever-so-pleasant smile creeping across her wide lips, she looked directly into Roy's eyes.

"A rest room?" Roy asked.

"Certainly. This executive section has a rest room, but we prefer that you use the one off the foyer in that direction." Roy turned in the direction the young lady was pointing. He had tried that area without any luck. To Roy it was a huge maze. He thanked the girl and started back down the hall from where he had emerged, when a purple-robed woman-- not old, not young, maybe fortyish, Roy thought, nodded to Roy, then quickly stopped beside the girl in blue. "Sarah, I need your help at the desk. It seems there is too much for Miriam to handle by herself with all the guests today."

Roy began to walk back toward the foyer, then stopped. The two women had exited through a side door and were gone. He whirled around and decided he would find the  rest room on that particular wing since no one else was around to stop him. He hoped there were no more compound ushers, security people, or whatever they were, to stop him. He had to go.

He knew he was in the executive wing, a private, off-limits location for a visitor. It made no difference. The tinted skylights on the arched ceiling above him cast an amber glow on the white walls. He had searched the wing to the right and found no rest room. He had used one near the dining hall in Gateway's main building of the compound earlier in the day. One of the youths thought there was a rest room at the north end of the building, but Roy hadn't found it. There had to be one somewhere in the area. A diabetic with special needs, he was desperate by now. He rushed past several light, oak-stained double doors—executive offices, no doubt—alert to any door that might lead to a rest room. It crossed Roy's mind that the Grand Oracle Josiah must have a rather elaborate office somewhere in this wing. But the pressing need for him at the moment was a rest room—fast.

In the hallway at the center of the wing, Roy spotted a door he hoped was the right one. As he reached for the doorknob, the door opened inwardly and a young man, maybe 20 years old, red headed and wearing jeans, came out pushing a cleaning cart, complete with a mop. Roy stood back while the young man moved past him with a nod, then disappeared down the hall. Roy grabbed the slowly closing door. All right! It was a rest room. At last, relief.

He quickly glanced about the shiny, tiled room. To the left was a commode slightly visible beyond the stall's door. The three basins were made of gleaming white porcelain with a distinctive design, as if they had been hand crafted. The fixtures appeared to be gold plated, elegant against the black-veined, marble countertop, definitely a notch above the usual public facilities. He rushed into the stall and latched the door behind him. The booth was fitted with a solid core, three-quarter-high door. It extended from the floor up six feet and from there was open to the ceiling.

Empty. Great!

As he relieved himself, he heard clicking sounds. It sounded as if someone were unlocking the door. No, it was at least two people. He could hear their muffled voices. It dawned on Roy that this must be the executive rest room. He listened as the men entered. They spoke to one another as they walked across the tile floor at the far end—low tones, quiet yet husky sounds.

Roy froze.

He reasoned that if they had a key to what seemed to be a very private rest room, it followed they had to be high-ups in Gateway.

Roy slumped down as he sat on the stool. Drawing silent breaths, he hoped to avoid detection. He was irritated at the whole situation. *So what if he had encroached on the territory of the elite? They should have provided more readily available facilities.* Yet Roy's sensitive personality was not suited for this sort of encounter, and he was still concerned about being found out. He didn't want to embarrass himself by being discovered in a rest room he was now certain was reserved for executives with keys.

Chagrined, Roy could imagine all sorts of scenarios, none of them pleasant. If they discovered him, they might think he was snooping around the executive wing and had ducked into the rest room to avoid detection. Oh well. What could they do anyway, sue him? It wasn't that. He didn't want the confrontation.

Roy became increasingly uncomfortable as he realized that one of the voices was definitely that of the Grand Oracle Josiah—head man. The aura around the Grand Oracle Josiah invaded Roy's thoughts. He had met the great man at lunch in the dining hall earlier. The Oracle had a unique husky voice, and his eyes had been partially hidden behind expensive, gold-rimmed, tinted glasses. He had shaken hands with Roy and there was something strange about the religious leader that had troubled Roy. A shiver swept over his body. He would be glad to leave this stark building complex and head home to Provo.

Stephen and Dr. Polk had urged Roy to join a group of touring journalists for several reasons. Certainly, they wanted to get some idea of what the Oracle Josiah's impression of such a holy city might be. But they also wanted to determine how the world saw the Second Coming and how their depiction of the event would dovetail with the scriptures.

He silently waited, still seated on the toilet, forced to eavesdrop. The conversation was fragmented, like that of two old friends who did not bother to finish statements but rushed from topic to topic.

"I don't like this . . . "

"It's good PR . . . "

Roy tried to fill in the gaps of the disjointed conversation. He heard the other voice, the person he had seen in the dining room, say something about an accident.

Now the Oracle spoke clearly. He had turned away from where he was standing and spoke in Roy's direction. His voice was deep and raspy but had a resounding, almost compelling, rhythmic tone, certainly unique. Roy caught his breath as he listened.

"I hate these executions, Reuben. How many must we have to convince our people that they have committed to remain loyal?"

Yes, it was definitely the Oracle speaking. *Executions? What was he talking about?* An uneasy feeling swept over Roy, the same feeling he had experienced at lunch when he shook hands with the Oracle.

"I'll set up the accident after dark. I'll get Jeremiah and Lot to help me," said the other man, the one the Oracle called Reuben. Then Roy heard the urinal flush.

"Good. You know what to do," the Oracle replied.

"Use a Jeep and see that it rolls at least a thousand feet down Mirage Mountain, right?"

Roy heard them cross the white tile floor and stop. He remained absolutely still. He kept his feet from moving. No sound. Cold sweat trickled down his body. They were talking about executing someone . . . killing someone in a Jeep. . . . Naw. They couldn't be serious. Not murder. Surely he hadn't heard right.

"As I said, I gain no pleasure from this sort of activity," the Oracle repeated calmly.

Roy could detect no sorrow in the man's voice. He silently shook his head in bewilderment. That anyone could calmly plan to kill or dispose of another human was totally foreign to him. Roy wanted desperately to block out the voices coming through the closed door of the stall. It was as if he had intruded on an intimate conversation between lovers or had overheard the plotting of war by ministers of state.

"The kid was good with assault weapons. I helped train him," Reuben replied with pride. His voice was higher and sharper in tone than the Oracle's. "But he may have been headed for the sheriff's office in one of the compound vehicles when we intercepted him outside the gates."

"The thing I hate most is the way we have to carry out these trials. If it weren't for those stupid journalists here for the day, we could have whisked his body to the mountains and notified the authorities before dark. The longer his body remains in the cave, the greater the risk. Some sharp coroner is going to place the time of death earlier than we want it to appear. Besides, they'll want to know what he was doing driving a Jeep in the steep mountains after dark."

"Patrolling," Reuben shot back. "We'll tell them we've beefed up our security efforts at night. Patrolling our borders, that's all. What's wrong with that? I'll let the word get around that Seth is out patrolling the south ridge this evening. Late tonight when he fails to report in, we'll send a party out to search for him. They'll find that he drove off a cliff in the dark."

"Too bad we have to destroy a Jeep. I need all my vehicles. At least it's covered by insurance. . . . But we have to deal decisively with those who break the code."

"Everything will be handled as usual," Reuben assured the Oracle. "I know how to take care of these things."

"Yeah. I hope so. But there will still be an investigation."

Roy could hear water splashing into the basin and the clatter of the paper towel dispenser. Was that the door opening? He desperately hoped so. They must be leaving. He could hear diminishing footsteps.

Stunned, Roy's heart was pounding and the perspiration building. It was all so . . . so . . . surreal. This couldn't be happening. This was no longer a matter of embarrassment; he had overheard a plot, a cover-up to murder.

Maybe he hadn't heard them right. He hadn't gotten in on the early part of their conversation. How could he arrive at such a conclusion based on eavesdropping? But he knew deep inside that he had heard correctly.

Roy's personal concern went beyond the death of this guy named Seth. What if they learned he had been in the room while they talked so freely? He wondered what they would do if they knew he had overheard their conversation. It could mean his own life.

* * *

Not a month ago, Brenda had left college with high hopes that kept her at a wild-horse pace. She had come all the way to Wyoming in an effort to meet the Oracle and consented to learn more about his group. She was elated, sure that she was actually encountering the ultimate religious experience. Her escorts had taken her directly to an enormous cavern that reminded her of the inside of the giant Astrodome in Houston. It was large enough to house not only the tarp-covered vehicles the Oracle had acquired, but also accommodated a couple of prefabricated buildings that served as the nerve center of the compound. Those who had access to the cave comprised a select few, and they were chiefly the cadre of security. Most of the youth at Gateway had not been inside since completing their indoctrination.

The communications center inside the cave linked Gateway to the world through telephones, computer networks and the latest classified security systems in the federal government. Such elaborate electronic equipment came at a high price, but the Oracle had dreams of cloning Gateway throughout America and other select parts of the world. In his grand plan it would require a ten-year program to achieve, but succeed he would. After all, he was building the new world for his God. No servant of God had ever achieved in so short a time a framework for the City of God. What a splendid moment it had been when Brenda knelt before the Oracle and received his assurance that she had made a wise choice for her future.

Her instructor, Mother Martha, came through the door to Brenda's small room inside the prefabricated building within the cave. When Brenda began her training, she had not concerned herself with such mundane things as freedom to come and go as she chose. Inside the cave, deep within one of the side tunnels, was a brick-laid path she had been taken down to the tropical pond, there to bask in the delights of water and sand with two other college girls who had arrived a few days before Brenda. The smaller cavern sheltered a pond of sparkling warm water fed from hot springs deep inside the mountain. It was banked with pure white sand that had been trucked in from beaches south of Carmel in California. Banana, mango, and orange trees growing around the pond were nourished by imported soil. Massive plant lights gave the tropical pool all the ambiance of the coast of Tahiti.

At first Brenda was unaware that Mother Martha, who acted as therapist, was injecting heroin between her toes as she gently massaged Brenda's body, rubbing a topical anesthetic along the soft skin between her toes to mask any pain associated with the injections. The massage and injection usually followed Brenda's swim in the tropical pool. Soon thereafter, Brenda began to beg Martha to inject the magic potion into her veins. But, following methods, Martha held out until Brenda was screaming for the next shot.

Now Brenda lay on her metal frame bed, begging for Mother Martha to come. Beginning the evening before, she had tried to open her bedroom door, but discovered for the first time that it was locked. By midnight she was pounding and screaming at the door, shouting for Mother Martha to bring her the stuff. She was aware it was a drug of some sort, a drug she now required. She cried out for the therapist over and over again, but she didn't come.

By late afternoon, when Brenda had not slept since the day before—she was unable to relax or do anything but beg—Martha came through the door to Brenda's small room inside the prefabricated building. Brenda grabbed her like a child teetering at the edge of a cliff, terrified that Mother Martha would leave without giving her the needle. As Brenda held tight to Martha's blouse, face in her face, sweat poured from her temples. Her eyes were wide, her teeth grinding. "I need it, Mother Martha," she whimpered. Martha had instructed Brenda to call her by her Gateway title, Mother Martha. It was the Oracle who insisted that all occupants of Gateway use biblical names.

"Mother, Mother Martha. Give it to me. I need it now!" The falsetto voice hardly sounded like Brenda—Brenda, the daughter of Stephen and Anney, the sister of Todd, the honor student of Lafayette High, the A student at Redlands, the jilted girlfriend of Max. This always-in-control person was now groveling in the depths of drug dependency. Her whole life now centered around a fix. Her entire mental attitude had become one of survival until the next injection.

"My, my, Rachel," Mother Martha said to Brenda, applying Brenda's Gateway name, "all you needed to do was ask. Lie down. I have it right here."

Brenda released her grip on Martha, whirled about, and in one leap lay supine upon the bed, gripping the mattress as she eyed the woman who held the needle and syringe in her hand. Relief. Blessed relief would come in minutes, maybe sooner. *How could she have been so misguided? What had come over her to allow herself to consent to enter the Gateway order?* She searched for answers as she tossed about on the cot. *How would she ever make contact with her family that now seemed comprised of the most ideal people in the world? Somehow she would escape. Somehow.*

\* \* \*

At last Roy heard the delayed click of the restroom door closing, then silence. Good, they were gone. Relief flooded Roy's thoughts for a moment, but only a moment. He knew he had to get out and fast . . . but not too fast. Realizing the two men could linger in the hall, Roy waited. His emotions built, bristling to send him flying from the premises. Still he waited. Two minutes passed, then three. It seemed like hours before he summoned the courage to open the stall door. He moved lightly to the rest room door and opened it a crack to check the hall in both directions. Immensely relieved that the hall was empty and that his path to the north end of the wing and the location of the exit door was clear, he sprang into the hall and moved like a gazelle toward the exit sign.

As he rounded the corner to the alcove where the door was beckoning, Roy came face to face with a young man with orange-red hair. Roy saw with a start that it was the same fellow who had been cleaning the rest room a few minutes earlier. He wasn't nearly as tall as Roy. He was thin, with a frightened look on his pale face. He stepped in front of Roy, preventing him from reaching the door that led outside.

Roy stood frozen before this young man. He was already wound up by the nightmare in the rest room. Panic filled his whole body. He *had* to get out of there. He tried to step around the boy but was blocked a second time.

"Wait . . . listen," the young man whispered urgently. "I have to get out of here."

"You what?" Roy was confused. He thought the guy was trying to take him prisoner.

"You've got to help me! Take me with you."

Roy studied the boy's eyes. He saw desperation there. But he was desperate too.

"What are you talking about? I have nothing to do with anything around here." Roy tried to keep his voice from shaking. "Let me tell you straight: If you tried to leave with me, we would both be in deep trouble. I'm the wrong guy to ask."

Roy understood only too well why anyone would be scared out of his wits in this place after what he had overheard. He was ready to bolt the place himself.

Roy shook his head firmly. "I'm sorry, but I can't help you."

"You mean you won't help me," the boy argued.

"I said I can't." Roy began shoving the youth aside. As he reached for the door handle, the redhead grabbed his sleeve and held on.

"Hey, man, hands off," Roy hissed under his breath. "I said I can't help you."

"If they find out what I heard, they may kill me for what I know," said the boy, clearly pleading for his life.

Roy narrowed his eyes. Moments ago the same thought had crossed his own mind.

"Kill you? Why?" *Good grief! Were they going to execute him, too?*

The young man clenched his straight white teeth and begged, "Listen, one way or the other, I'm out of here. . . . I need a contact on the outside. Won't you just give me your phone number? *Please!* You don't know what it's like in here."

Roy peered more closely at the boy. He had a vivid understanding of the situation, but feared that he might do the kid more harm than good.

"My . . . uh . . . my phone number?" he stammered. "Uh . . . I live out of state. It won't do you any good."

"Please!"

Terrified as he was, Roy's heart went out to the youth. He reached into his shirt pocket, took out his pen and the pad he had been writing on during the tour, and dashed off his phone number. For a moment he was tempted to give a phony number. Then he put himself in the youth's place and wrote out the correct number to his condo in Provo, Utah. The youth grabbed it as soon as Roy wrote the last digit.

Roy pushed open the door, turned back toward the young redhead, and asked, "What's your name? I'll need to know if you call."

"I'll call . . . unless I'm dead. They changed my name to Daniel here at Gateway. But my real name is . . . "

The door sucked shut from the hydraulic force of the unit overhead before Roy could hear his real name. Did it matter? He was headed for freedom and home. Roy drew in the fresh Wyoming air, his first deep breath since his harrowing experience began a few minutes ago.

The journalists he had come with were boarding the chartered bus. He moved to the bus with long strides and climbed the two steps to its interior and what he hoped was safety. The diesel engine of the bus was idling—a good sound, a sound of freedom. Roy wanted out of this glorified hell hole, and now.

\* \* \*

Chief of security, Reuben stood in the Oracle's inner office when his small cell phone rang softly. He unfolded it and punched the button. "Yeah, Reuben here. What's up?"

"Oh, chief. Sorry to bother you," the voice on the phone replied, "but you asked me to report all activity with the journalists that looked even slightly out of the ordinary. I think you'd better come over to security control and check out one of the tapes that our executive hallway monitor recorded a few minutes ago."

The film offered proof enough for Reuben, who had rushed as quickly as his forty-something, out-of-shape body would carry him across the main hall to security control, a large room in the main structure. He watched the surveillance tape in angry silence as the youthful security man replayed the scene on a large screen at the back of the console. The color monitor had picked up Roy slipping into the rest room when the kid with housekeeping left it swinging wide open. The housekeeper hadn't turned around, hadn't noticed Roy grab the door, then slip inside. It was a rest room that required a key, reserved for the few. That wasn't at issue. Reuben knew very well that what he and the Oracle had discussed inside that room was highly sensitive information that could not escape the compound. The time recorded on the tape verified Roy did not emerge from the rest room until ten minutes later, *after* he and the Oracle had entered and exited. There was no mistake. The tape clearly showed the fellow slipping into the rest room, he and Josiah going in, going out, then this fellow going out. His face grim, Reuben reflected on the implications of the situation. He realized the guy had remained in the rest room while he and the Oracle spoke of the execution. This gawky young man in the turtleneck had to be stopped.

Reuben grabbed his cell phone, punched a button, waited impatiently for a response, then shouted, "Has the bus with those journalists left the compound?" If he had bothered to look up at the monitor on the extreme right, he could have seen that the bus was approaching the main gate to exit the premises but had not cleared the compound yet.

"The bus is here at the gate," the guard responded. "Shall I stop it?"

"Yes, stop it!" Reuben pulled the mouthpiece tight to his lips. "Now listen carefully. Don't just go storming on board. Step into the bus and very politely ask the fellow in a blue turtleneck—he's tall and thin—to accompany you off the bus. Got it? You are to detain him. Do it. I want him detained; I want to speak to him. Let the bus go through the gate. Tell the driver you'll be transporting the guy back to Jackson. Okay?"

"What's he going to say when I ask him to stay behind?"

"Just detain him. Be smooth about it. Now go! Get him off that bus. You hear me? Take him off the bus and hold him there at the gate house until I get there." Reuben clipped the phone to his belt and moved as fast as he could toward the gate.

\* \* \*

Roy watched the snappy, uniformed guard make his way along the aisle of the bus, scrutinizing each passenger. He was tall, blond, probably early twenties. Roy tensed and lowered his eyes. He knew who the guard was after: It had to be him. The starched uniform stopped at Roy's seat and leaned across Burton, his journalist friend, who occupied the seat on the aisle. The spiffy guard spoke politely.

"Sir, I have been asked to have you step into the gate house for a moment. Our head of security would like to speak with you. Please follow me."

Every eye in the bus was fixed on Roy.

But Roy had already made up his mind. He was not leaving the safety of the group. "No! I'd rather not meet with anyone," Roy shot back. "I'm staying right here."

"Please, sir, it will only take a minute. Our chief of security asked me to detain you."

Roy refused to budge from his seat. Burton turned to look closely at Roy, who had turned white. Something was not right.

Burton spoke up. "Didn't you hear him, buddy? He said no, so back off!"

The guard glanced at Burton, whose face was in his, and said, "Sir, this is not your affair. Please don't interfere."

"Interfere be damned," Burton shouted. "He's my assistant, and I say he's not going anywhere he chooses not to go."

The guard was about to argue when shouts went up from the journalists surrounding the midsection of the bus. "He doesn't want to talk to anyone." . . . "He doesn't have to do anything he doesn't want to." . . . "Leave him alone."

Amid the hubbub someone pulled up a Camcorder and began filming. Another took flash photos. A newspaper reporter got out of her seat to inspect the name tag on the guard's khaki uniform. Another shouted, "How do you spell your last name? Is it with a G or a C? I can't see. Sure want to get it right when I file this story." The tone of the journalists was light. No one took the matter seriously. What a joke to think a single guard was capable of removing anyone from the bus. Not likely, not if he refused to go.

Roy could see that none of the journalists, except perhaps his seat companion Burton, thought much of what was happening. To this hardened bunch of reporters it was a minor skirmish. From snatches of conversation Roy had heard during lunch, he knew a couple of these fellows had covered the Gulf War and others the Rwanda uprising. This young guard must have looked to them like a grade-school crossing guard telling an adult to step back onto the curb.

In the heart of the commotion, a loud voice thundered through the interior of the bus. It was the commanding voice of head of the security, a voice Roy recognized at once. It was chillingly familiar. The burly man at the front of the bus raised his hands to signal silence. He spoke loud enough for everyone to hear.

"Ladies and gentlemen, there has been a slight misunderstanding, and we need this young man to come with us for a moment," Reuben boomed, locking his eyes on Roy. "We will let the bus pass through, and one of our people will see that the gentleman is transported back to Jackson as soon as we have asked him a few questions."

Again cameras were activated and reporters began to do what they did best—cover breaking news, no matter how lame it appeared. "It looks like the name on your tag is Reuben, is that right?" came the voice of a pudgy reporter in the front seat. He reached up and pulled on Reuben's brown shirt sleeve to get his attention. "Tell us, Reuben, . . . what did the guy do, lift some silver-ware?" Roars of laughter filled the bus.

"Please, please, . . . all of you. It is my job to handle matters of security. Don't be rude."

"Rude, hell," the man at his elbow persisted. "I'm looking for a story; I sure haven't found one here today. We've been interviewing zombies. Maybe something worth reporting has actually happened, and all I want are the details."

"I ask you, ladies and gentlemen, please remain in your seats and do not get involved."

"Involved? Involved?" the journalist persisted. "If one of us is involved, we are all involved. You can't just come on board like some Nazi and make demands. What has this guy done?"

The chorus of voices began again. Reuben was drowned out. He knew there was no way he could remove the young man from the bus without an unpleasant scene. The journalists were no longer bantering and having sport at the expense of Reuben; they were turning mean. Reuben made a decision. He held up his hands again and asked everyone to please calm down. When relative silence came over the interior of the bus, he spoke.

"All right. I'm sorry for the delay—not a big deal. It appears this man does not want to cooperate with us. I'm sorry this visit has ended on a sour note." Reuben turned and lowered himself from the bus. He was concerned with what he knew Roy had overheard. As he stepped to the pavement, he nodded curtly to the driver to proceed, and with a snappy, military stride he walked toward the gate house. Moments later the gate opened and the bus drove through. Roy turned in his seat and looked through the window in time to see the man, Reuben, speaking rapidly on his cell phone.

As the bus sped along the picturesque Jackson Hole area, Roy sat in rigid silence, shocked by all that had happened so quickly. A horde of questions were fired at him from all corners of the bus, but even the good-natured badgering by the journalists couldn't persuade him to respond. Out of fear he remained silent. Silent because he didn't know what else to do. *Keep it to yourself. Don't say anything until you're certain what to say.* He was a master at silence. He had had a lifetime of training.

Burton had been with Roy for the past two days and could see the man was not about to talk. Give him time. Burton was certain that at the right moment, maybe not until they were on the bus traveling home tomorrow, would Roy divulge anything about what happened. He would make certain they sat together on the trip back to Salt Lake City. Burton was sometimes a patient man. Besides, he wanted the story to himself. Whatever it was that Roy was concealing might make interesting copy, a sort of footnote on the visit to Gateway. Perhaps it would lend a personal touch of excitement and intrigue.

\* \* \*

The chilled air at Salt Lake City International stung Katherine's cheeks as she stood with Samuel and Brad awaiting the airport limousine that would shuttle them to Provo. Darkness had kept trying to invade the landscape as the two flew west from Kansas City. Now the white lights that circled the main path of taxis, buses, and crowding cars sent white light across the waiting travelers. Katherine realized for the third time in as many hours that she was not as young as she pretended to be. The time zones and her body clock were out of sync, and every cell was shouting for timeout.

"I don't intend to see tomorrow morning. If you call, wake me after lunch, Samuel, honey."

Samuel nodded, his attention drawn to the airport limo that rounded the curve and began slowing to pick up those commuting to Provo.

# Chapter 5

A year ago Stephen and Anney would have sat at the kitchen table hovering over a steaming cup of coffee. That had changed. Now, seated in their kitchen, they sat looking at one another with two small glasses of orange juice separating them. Little else separated the two these days.

Stephen seldom went through his day without counting his attachment to Anney as his greatest achievement. At times his thoughts caused him to stop dead still and say to himself, *I almost lost her.* This morning, gloomy as the skies were through the wide kitchen window at their river-bottom home, plans dominated the conversation. Except for their concerns for the whereabouts of their daughter Brenda, they were positive, grateful, and in love with each other.

"I have a couple of things I want to talk to you about before I go meet with Samuel," Stephen said quietly as he looked at the slender, lightly-made-up face of the woman he adored. Stephen had known when he met Anney over twenty years ago at Berkeley that she would always be a child of nature. Still, her skin showed only very slight lines at the corners of the eyes. They were hardly visible. She looked thirty. Anney could still wear her hair to her shoulders and not be concerned that she looked as if she were clinging to her youth without success.

"What is it?" Anney asked, equally quiet in her response.

"You know, honey, we're going to be sealed in the temple in a week." He referred to an upcoming session in the temple and the sealing that would follow. Over the past six weeks they had taken the ward's temple preparedness course. The bishop had interviewed them and commented that he felt they were worthy to receive their temple recommends for the sealing session to take place in the Provo Temple. Todd, their nineteen-year-old son, was granted a recommend to go into a sealing room and be sealed to his parents. The only flaw that Anney and Stephen had already discussed at least a half a dozen times was their longing to have their daughter, Brenda, with them. It was not possible. Not only was she not a member, but she was supposedly off somewhere with a group of young people trying out a new lifestyle. And where she was they hadn't a clue.

Anney squeezed Stephen's unusually long fingers for his slightly less than six-foot frame. They were strong hands that Anney loved to feel touching her. Anney answered, "And I can hardly wait to be there."

"The thing I want to say is . . . well, how much you mean to me." Stephen studied Anney's features carefully. "I never dreamed I could fall for you a second time."

Anney looked puzzled.

Stephen quickly explained, "While I was shaving this morning, the thought that I almost lost you last year struck me so forcefully that I had to set down my razor and shake my head as I looked at myself in the mirror."

"Stephen, oh Stephen," Anney replied with that almost exasperated grin on her lips that Stephen had come to know so well, "that is old history. I don't know why you let yourself dwell on our months of desperately clinging to the hope that the worst time of our lives would end. It ended. It's behind us now. Surely you know it is." Anney referred to the bitter months after Stephen joined the Church and she continued to work with her father in his televangelic ministry that almost caused their divorce, though even at that time they loved each other dearly.

"I know this much: I would have crawled to wherever you were and laid prostrate in the dirt outside your door to beg for your love. Really, I would have." Stephen pulled back and placed both hands on the edge of the polished oak table top and shook his head as he studied Anney's face. "I can't believe how close we came to destroying the most precious relationship the world has ever known. I mean it. I love you. And I truly want you for eternity." A wide smile crossed Stephen's full, lightly tanned face that, now that winter was setting in, was returning to its natural reddish appearance. He still had that boyish flare to his wide eyes and full lips. The strawberry-blond hair had thinned and gave him the appearance of a 45-year-old man, which he was, but otherwise youth clung to his features like the last leaves of fall on an oak tree. "My talk is pretty heavy stuff for this time of the day, don't you think?"

"Don't spoil it, sweetheart. I love it." Anney reached all the way across the table and once again squeezed Stephen's hand. "I just love it."

* * *

Roy had slept little. He awoke sleepy this morning with a startled recollection of what he had overheard. The tragedy of what he had stumbled upon left him numb and confused, and the dilemma of what to do and whether to make it known whirled around in his churning thoughts, thoughts that stirred him to the bone. He knew in his heart he did not want to discuss what he had heard with anyone but Dr. Polk, the one man he admired most in all his training these past couple of years. He remained silent. Not anyone. How could he trust such information to any of those he was with? They were all strangers. Burton he had known only a few days. He wished desperately that he had not come on this trip. He didn't need to see Josiah's Gateway for ideas; he could design a futuristic display of the New Jerusalem without a firsthand impression by some wacko. He certainly had an impression all right, an impression of horror and fear.

Now he stood shaving in his shorts at the bathroom sink in his room at the Jackson Hole Inn, listening to an early news broadcast from the television set in the other room. The local anchorwoman had covered the world and the national scene, then after a commercial had switched to the local news. Suddenly, Roy's eyes glanced up to stare at his image in the mirror. He could see the color seep from his face. It was not just the note of sorrow in the newscaster's voice that drew Roy's attention and pulled him from the bathroom to stand in front of the television, shaving cream still slathered on one side of his face. He was stunned by her words.

She had been saying, "Late last night in the eastern mountains, local rescue teams from the sheriff's department retrieved the body of a 21-year-old youth who apparently careened off the mountain road to his death in a Jeep he was driving. Details are still sketchy, but Deputy Lewis of the sheriff's department informed K-News that the Jeep rolled several times, crushing the victim, finally coming to rest five hundred feet down a ravine." Roy focused on the announcer's lips as she said, "The sheriff's department has asked that we withhold the name of the victim until the family can be notified. We have learned, however, that the victim was a member of the controversial Gateway religious group, and that the accident took place on a ridge three miles from the compound. . . . In other news, . . . "

Roy blocked out the announcer's voice, put his hands to his temples, and shook his head. Suddenly he knew for sure that murder had been committed at Gateway. And yet . . . should he tell someone what he had heard? All his life he had kept things to himself. He was never strong in verbal skills; he had never considered himself strong in any personality traits for that matter. Among his peers at college in Boston, he had at times been the target of off-the-wall kidding. Socially he was a nerd, and he knew it. He was too bright not to see that.

Roy saw himself as not simply shy, but awkward too; thin, even gaunt and bony. His physical makeup, combined with his socially insecure personality, projected an image that wasn't really him deep down inside. To those who were able to penetrate his protective shell, Roy was warm and had cultivated a sense of humor. At Harvard he was the brightest in his class, if sheer testing proved anything. However, he never took advantage of his genius to best anyone. In fact, he seldom asserted himself lest he be noticed. That was Roy.

This fear of being singled out seemed to compel Roy to hold things in. He was doing it now as he debated with himself whether or not to tell Burton what he had heard. No, not Burton. Who then? Dr. Polk?

Contrary to what others thought of Roy, Dr. Polk, his aging, wheelchair-bound boss and best friend, considered him the most valuable assistant he could possibly have. Those personality traits that kept girls at bay were assets to Polk. If nothing else, Roy was focused. Above all, Dr. Polk saw Roy as dedicated to the Book of Mormon Center and its success.

Young Roy Carver was without question the most skilled programmer and electronic designer for the Book of Mormon Center that Peter Polk, Professor Emeritus of BYU, could have discovered. At the Center, contractors had installed and readied the hardware, all the mechanized apparatus. Then, with meticulous skill, Roy had taken over and now maintained the day-to-day electronic operations.

He saved the foundation (which had been created three years before by Polk and his deceased friend, Thomas Kline) tens of thousands of dollars that would otherwise have been spent to hire an entire crew to program and maintain the various sections of the popular Center. The Center had been created to offer visitors a bird's-eye view—through video, miniature relief land masses, and wonderful diorama depictions of the Book of Mormon culture—of the layout of the Book of Mormon lands.

Roy decided that he would hold off mentioning anything about what had happened until he spoke with Dr. Polk and got his input.

* * *

In his quest to uncover current thinking on the city that the leader of the compound dubbed Gateway, the grand city to be constructed before the Second Coming, Burton had heard of Dr. Polk and his Book of Mormon Center. Actually, it was Burton's editor who knew of Polk and sent him to take a look at the Book of Mormon Center in preparation for his scheduled visit to Gateway in Wyoming. It was all part of his ongoing research for a television news special to put together a segment about religious Utopian societies, historical and contemporary. It would be a regional special originating in Salt Lake City.

Roy had escorted Burton around the Book of Mormon Center and shown him the entire attraction that had been created to highlight the geography and culture of the Book of Mormon—all inside the cavern of an old building that had once been a supermarket.

It was Polk who had asked Burton if Roy could tag along as an assistant so that he could view the so-called Gateway in Wyoming. The invitation to the compound was restricted to journalists. But as Burton's assistant for a day, Roy could get a glimpse of the highly publicized Gateway—technically as a reference point for creating the depiction of the New Jerusalem in Provo, but in reality to satisfy Polk's curiosity. Burton had gone along with the idea and Roy had promised to be careful. With his photographic skills, Roy would be useful to the Salt Lake-based newsman; Burton had brought along a camcorder to do a preliminary layout of the projected series, at least in the initial stages. Roy put on a convincing show when he filmed Burton descending the steps of the chartered bus. The only real hitch up to this point came when compound security insisted that all cameras and filming equipment remain on the bus. Too bad.

Roy caught his mind whirling once again. He felt that the reality of what he had heard would never leave his mind. Never!

*Why? Why had he become a party to such horror?* The compound security suspected he knew something. Somehow Gateway security knew he had been in that rest room. It hit him why. At the Book of Mormon Center he had personally set up the camera monitoring system to guard the Center around the clock. Of course, a television monitor had picked up his entrance into the rest room and his exit as well. The security guard had been concentrating on the main lobby monitor where there were a number of journalists at the front desk asking for the membership roster. He missed seeing Roy's entrance and exit. But by reviewing the tapes, Gateway security knew that he had been in a stall when the two executives were in the rest room.

# Chapter 6

Jeremiah sat hunched over the wheel of his Ford F-150 pickup as he observed what was happening from his rear-view mirror. He learned by cell phone in code from Reuben that the lanky fellow he was shadowing was named Roy. He could see Roy standing near the charter bus with his bag in his left hand and extending his right hand to another fellow that Jeremiah didn't know. He surmised they were saying goodbye to one another. Jeremiah had watched his speed while tailing the charter bus all the way from Jackson Hole, making sure he remained as far back along the freeway as two miles, still keeping the bus in sight at all times. He had been trained by the best in vehicular shadowing. When the charter bus pulled into the Flying J truck stop outside of Brigham City, Jeremiah waited at the side of the frontage road, which was void of traffic. And while he waited, he got out of the pickup and quickly replaced his Wyoming plates with Idaho plates. It would be hard to trace those bogus plates from Idaho. He had jumped through hoops to conceal their origin—they had come off a demolished pickup that he bought from the owner through a false name.

It had been a smooth ride for Jeremiah from the freeway off ramp to downtown Salt Lake, ending up at the DoubleTree Hotel. When the bus stopped under the portico, Jeremiah pulled into a ten-minute parking space thirty feet from the bus.

He watched as the group of journalists disembarked from the bus. Finally, Roy stepped off and retrieved his bag. Jeremiah focused most of his attention on Roy's actions. He knew from cryptic conversation on the cell phone out of Jackson Hole that Roy lived and worked in Provo, so he would be taking some other form of transportation from Salt Lake City—maybe his own car. Reuben had furnished Jeremiah with the model and license number of Roy's van, which Reuben had pulled off the computer after searching the Utah State auto records.

Jeremiah lost visual contact when Roy moved across the portico to the underground parking terrace of the Double Tree. *He's going after his van.*

Jeremiah remained in his truck and waited. Roy couldn't slip from his grasp; there was just one exit and he had that covered.

As Jeremiah kept an eye focused on the scene, he noticed the other fellow who had said goodbye to Roy. The guy was moving up alongside the truck to the driver's side. Jeremiah tracked his every movement. Then he stopped beside the pickup's door.

*What the hell's going on?* wondered Jeremiah as he turned to meet the man's eyes through the window.

He motioned for Jeremiah to lower his window. He wanted to share something with him. Jeremiah reluctantly complied with the sign language request.

"Yes?"

The intruder swung his head toward the rear of the truck bed and said aloud. "I see you have a Twin Falls license plate. Are you from there? I was born and raised in Twin Falls. My name's Thom Burton; my dad has a farm there."

Jeremiah shook his head. "No, I'm not. This is a leased truck," he lied.

Burton glanced up to the double K.C. beams on the cab roof and said, "Why two sets of beams on top?"

"I have no idea. It came that way from Avis. I guess for rough country. It's a four-by-four." Jeremiah was cool in his response. Burton got the message that he didn't want to talk.

"Well, have a good one." Burton felt foolish for asking the guy. *How lame can you get?* he wondered to himself. He hated to look stupid.

"Oh, well. Sorry I bothered you. Just thought I'd ask. You know, every time I see 2T on an Idaho plate, I generally ask the driver if he knows anybody I do. Sorry."

"No problem." Jeremiah rolled up the window and quickly surveyed the entrance to the underground garage. At that moment Jeremiah spotted Roy's mud-streaked van emerging from the terrace below. Roy inched slowly past Jeremiah and stopped before entering First West to proceed on to Provo.

It was Roy, all right. Jeremiah knew to fall in behind him as soon as Roy was a half-block down the street; experience cautioned against any abrupt moves. Part of vehicular shadowing involved slow movements and anticipation, like any hunting sport. He looked to his side, reached under the seat, and pulled up his Beretta before moving off. When he reached the signal, he pushed the gun back under the seat. He knew that this hit would not require a gun. The two ordinary plastic grocery bags he had also stuffed under the seat would do just fine. So far he had snuffed out two lives with bags. It was such a clean method of elimination.

* * *

It was an early supper night for Anney and Stephen. It had been a long day: Up early, meetings until late this afternoon, then moving boxes early this evening. Stephen was hungry. The two sat in the not-yet-decorated kitchen of their new home located in the river-bottom area of Provo, surrounded by boxes and odd pieces of furniture, things that Anney had not yet decided where to place. Unpacking and arranging treasured pieces in an orderly yet creative manner was not her thing in this life. She relied on Stephen and others to help.

As Stephen talked, Anney noticed how disinterested she was and thought how quickly she had begun to cut people off while they discussed mundane projects. He knew her deep concern about Brenda had completely engulfed her life, but the way to correct the situation seemed a mystery. Finally, Stephen stopped talking, too. The two sat silently eating the pasta she had picked up in the Smith's deli. It seemed easier lately to stop by a deli and grab prepared food than to fix a meal for two. *It hasn't always been this way,* she thought wistfully. With Brenda and Todd at home last summer, she had laid out regular meals and the family had loved it. She had always enjoyed cooking special dishes for her family, but lately . . . Anney had to admit that in some ways living with Stephen and no one else had its advantages. At least she didn't have as much kitchen clean-up to do.

"I enjoyed last night's dinner, didn't you?" Stephen asked, breaking the silence as he pressed his paper napkin to his chin to blot away the fettucini sauce. "Yeah, quite a change from elegant dining to a supper of take-out in this room full of boxes and me in my grubbies." He grinned teasingly. "But I don't mind," he hastened to add. "I doubt that I could live at that level of sophistication for very long. I'd hate to dress for every meal. I kinda like things casual. Don't you?"

"Sure. . . . are you trying to make me feel good about the way I feed you these days? Shaming me into old-fashioned cooking won't work. It's a lost cause." Anney kept up her end of the light banter. "I've looked forward to the simple life—just sort of kicking back the way we've done today."

"Me, too."

"Yeah? Don't try to kid me. You love those big family meals." Anney stood up and carried her paper plate to the sink, deposited her fork and glass, and turned to the refrigerator. "Would you like some ice cream? I bought your favorite . . . Vanilla Bean."

"Sure," Stephen replied, pushing his paper plate to the center of the table. "I'll need the extra jolt of sugar to move all those boxes in the garage and make room for one more car. Stacks of them are out there right now screaming for me to get with it." Stephen picked up his fork and turned it over in his hand as he spoke. "Honey, thanks for making this move easier than it would have been if you had resisted. I really appreciate you going along with it."

Anney nodded without comment.

Stephen and Anney Thorn had uprooted themselves from their Lafayette home in the East Bay Area of San Francisco and had moved to Provo so Stephen could pursue his work with Dr. Polk at the Book of Mormon Center.

Within the last year and a half, first Stephen, then Anney, and later their son, Todd, had all joined the Church. The Book of Mormon and key people in the Book of Mormon projects had helped the Thorns undergo a transformation of religious learning. Their whole spiritual reference to life had turned in a marvelous new direction. From Stephen's first encounter with the Book of Mormon on an estate in north San Diego to this very moment, he had continually experienced an intense training course in the gospel of Jesus Christ, and particularly in the Book of Mormon. Stephen had become so engrossed in the patterns of Book of Mormon prophecy and the new insights it offered that he had been ready to join the Church when he finished reading the Book of Mormon the first time.

It had now been a little over a year since he accepted the position as paid assistant to Dr. Polk. Stephen had helped develop the Book of Mormon Center situated off University Avenue in North Provo near the Brigham Young University stadium. He had come to understand how important the Book of Mormon was for members of the Church.

When Stephen and Anney made the decision about their future plans, it was either transfer to Provo and do a decent job of directing projects for the Book of Mormon Center, or stay in the Bay Area and take a new job. Anney agreed with Stephen, who was eager to continue with his work at the Center. It had taken some soul searching to leave the area where they had spent all twenty-two years of their married life, then to sell their house that Anney had so lovingly decorated over ten years ago, pack, and move. The Trust paid for the van that moved them from California to Utah. Their house in Lafayette sold for $400,000 (their equity was $150,000), while the home in the river bottoms in Provo at Pheasant Green cost $350,000, which they financed for $100,000 down. So Anney had some cash to decorate all over again, only this time she had the funds to do it right.

Of course, there was also her inheritance from her father, but she and Stephen had decided months ago to let those funds remain in their investment portfolio and to live off their own income, at least for the time being.

The week before, they had been in San Francisco in the financial district at their attorney's office, poring over the estate of the late Robert Moore, Anney's televangelist father, who had died months earlier. Part of the funds Anney's father had left to her were swallowed up in estate taxes and legal fees. Still, Anney and Stephen would come away with a tidy sum—several hundred thousand dollars. That was primarily money that Robert Moore's wealthy wife of a year, Katherine, had placed into his account to ease the financial burden of carrying out an ambitious evangelical television ministry, which the Reverend Moore was so gifted in maintaining.

Katherine had insisted that the money left in her late husband's estate was Anney's and Stephen's. She wanted nothing more than to see her stepdaughter and Stephen enjoy the funds for whatever needs they had. And they did have needs. Though Stephen was making $75,000 annually with the Book of Mormon project, it was good to have the additional funds to get resettled in Provo, and to make certain that their two children had sufficient money for their education. Their son, Todd, had already committed himself to leave on a Church mission the next summer when he finished his spring quarter at Utah Valley State College. He was living in an apartment with his best friend and fellow classmate, Max Williams. Todd was already enrolled in school when his parents decided to move to Provo. He never entertained the idea of moving in with them. They were only a couple of miles apart. It was cool to live off campus in student housing where he could stay out late if he decided to and have friends in for TV football on Monday nights without bothering his parents. There was nothing new about living without family for Max. Even though his street days were over, the harshness of life on the street had made its mark. He never quite felt that he was tied to anyone. The Thorns were the closest thing to family he knew, but, Max understood, there were limits to their affection.

Perhaps it was a persistent desire on the part of Max to be permanently connected to the Thorns as a son-in-law that had driven him to propose marriage to Brenda in the first place. Then reality had hit him on the yacht when he knew he wanted to serve a mission. "I should never have asked Brenda to marry me," Max had confided to his best friend Todd. "Your sister deserves a better life than I could ever give her."

Anney scooped up the empty plastic container from the deli as Stephen stood up, ready to return to the garage and to start bringing in more boxes marked for certain areas of the house. He noticed how short the days were in November. It was already dusk. This evening he knew he would work until his fingers were stiff and numb and his back ready to scream before he could drop into bed. He wanted to get the job over with, and there was no other way to get it done. The movers had stacked the boxes in the crowded garage. It was up to Stephen to move them to the various rooms of the house. Wouldn't you know both Todd and Max had classes tonight?

# Chapter 7

Legs feeling cramped, Roy crawled out of his vintage Toyota van and slammed the door behind him. It was dark now. Tired as he was, he had decided he should drop by the Book of Mormon Center and check his answering machine for business calls. He had tried to access his calls from a telephone booth as soon as the bus arrived in Salt Lake City, but something must have happened with the tape. All he heard was static. He wanted to know who had called the Center. He was expecting a recording crew from Los Angeles in the morning. Perhaps they had tried to reach him with a change of plans, he thought.

Roy pulled up to the section of the curb painted red with NO PARKING in white lettering on the surface of the concrete. The Center was closed for the evening with no classes scheduled. The parking lot was totally empty. In the blackness of night, the street lamps obscured the crazy-quilt tar patching of the twenty-year-old asphalt surface. Roy knew the only reason for the no parking section close to the Center was to accommodate deliveries and the unloading of tour groups, neither of which would be happening tonight, so there was no reason to park farther away.

It had been a long day for Roy; actually, a long three days. First the trip to Wyoming the day before, the lengthy visit to Gateway yesterday, then a poor night's rest and the long trip home, not to mention his harrowing experience in the rest room.

It wasn't the travel that wearied him. It was the weight on his mind of the death of the young man from the compound. Roy did not know how to ease his mind away from what he had overheard and was still undecided about where he should go with his information. He had already made up his mind to speak to Dr. Polk about his terrifying Gateway experience, but that would have to wait until morning. It was after nine now, and he knew Polk would be in bed—if not sleeping, at least reading and ready to fall asleep. Such news would only stir him up and perhaps rob him of a restful night. Polk needed all the rest he could get. A stroke had left the 72-year-old professor with reduced strength.

Roy thought the next person he ought to talk with was Stephen, if he couldn't speak to Dr. Polk. He had tried to reach Stephen at his new home and got the standard answering machine message. The Thorns were unpacking in their garage and could not hear the phone ringing. Roy left a message asking Stephen to call him when he got in. He told him on the recorder that he would be at the Center and had some vital information to share with him. Would he please call as soon as he got the message?

Now Roy wished he had called Stephen the evening before, or at least from the inn in Jackson Hole before he boarded the bus to return to Salt Lake City. But he hadn't, and he was puzzled as to why he hadn't. But then it was not the sort of thing you blurt out over the phone. What he knew needed to be discussed carefully and presented to the proper authorities. He would do it first thing in the morning. Or, if Stephen wanted to come to the Center, he would tell him tonight. Roy couldn't see how he could fall asleep anyway. He had dozed off a couple of times while he labored over his laptop on the bus coming back from Wyoming. Then he had nearly driven off the freeway at the Point of the Mountain when his eyes closed for a moment. He had caught the wheel and jerked the van back into the right-hand lane, where he had sense enough to drive. That had startled him so that he made it to the Center in Provo wide awake.

* * *

They had gathered earlier in the day at the Homestead Resort in the Heber Valley, twenty-eight miles from Provo. The group of authors and three Brigham Young University professors were already in the cozy dining room of the Homestead. Much of the light came flickering from large candles spread throughout the room. The fireplace, made of gray stone, roared with large logs of cherry wood. The atmosphere was one of congenial hosting, with several groups scattered about the room. It was not crowded.

Samuel followed the maître d' to the far end of the dining room. Plants blocked the view of the professors who had already begun their split pea soup. When the host, Bender, saw Samuel come striding behind the maître d', he arose, arms spread, and said loud enough for all to hear, "Sam, come in, please.

Come right over and take this seat we have reserved for you on my left. Come, my friend."

The entire group of a dozen people at the table turned as Bender welcomed this special participant. They were all smiles. Samuel started to explain that he had been delayed with several phone calls, then thought better of it. They really didn't care what his delay had been. He was here now and that was all that really mattered. If Katherine had been invited, he would have asked her to come along, but she hadn't. This was strictly a meeting of the minds on matters regarding the return of the Savior. Samuel already knew, as he took the high-backed, purple-velvet-seated chair and sat at the place that had been reserved for him, that everyone at the table was either a noted LDS author or a gifted lecturer on the subject at hand.

The gathering was the second of its kind that had been scheduled to meet and discuss current thinking on the coming of Christ. Samuel had been contacted by Bender over a week ago. He had told Samuel that he and the others who would attend were inviting three guest speakers, and would Samuel care to address such an august body of thinkers and writers? Samuel had conferred with Polk, and the two decided to accept the invitation. Bender had not been specific in just what he wanted Samuel to speak about, but Samuel knew it had something to do with his longtime research into events leading up to the Second Coming. Bender did indicate it ought to be in his realm of recent research.

* * *

With no experience in being followed, Roy had been easy prey for Jeremiah, whose pickup stayed fairly close to the van all the way to Provo.

Preoccupied as he was, Roy didn't see the truck glide to the curb with its lights off and stop a half-block from the Center's entrance. The man inside was hidden by the heavy shrubs that lined the south side of the lot.

Jeremiah waited a few minutes before getting out of his pickup. While he waited, he put a call through on his cell phone to Reuben at the compound. He wanted to know for certain that this person he was following should be "removed" from his list. Reuben understood the code. The words "remove" or "delete" meant the same thing—death to Roy. Reuben affirmed that Jeremiah's orders were to delete or remove Roy Carver.

Jeremiah got out of the pickup quietly, standing still for a few moments, looking carefully in all directions. He reached beneath the front seat and retrieved two ordinary tan plastic grocery bags, one inside the other, with the bold lettering Albertsons on both sides. He wadded them into a ball and stuffed them up his left sleeve. From the pocket of his Levis, he pulled out a small, black knife and checked it to be sure he had all the equipment he needed.

*  *  *

The small talk around the table was shop talk, naturally. Everyone, it seemed to Samuel, was eager to share his insights on when to expect the Second Coming. Strange speculation that this group indulged in since only the Father knows the exact time of the Second Coming. Samuel knew that around this particular table, this very evening, were the most outstanding lecturers and authors of the Church anywhere on the Second Coming, except, perhaps, General Authorities. Why shouldn't they speculate? It was their nature.

A dessert of fried ice cream and a soft German cookie completed the meal.

Bender stood at the head of the table and once again addressed the group made up of nine men and three women, all scholars to one degree or the other. Samuel knew most by name and two by sight. He had read the works on the Second Coming by each of the four writers in the group. He saw Caldwell at the far end of the table, a man in his sixties who was the first so-called contemporary author to have a best seller on prophecy. His book had been a major read in the Church for the past thirty-five years and was still going strong. Pity it was flawed when it came to what would have to transpire prior to the Second Coming. And what about Clawson, who stayed right on top of prophecy? He was also totally unaware of the key item all the writers had missed. Everyone had missed it. By diligent research, Samuel had found the key that would open the door to preparation for the Second Coming.

Bender rubbed his hands together as he continued to speak, "Brothers and Sisters, I would like to have us stay right here at the table and have Samuel Meyers take his forty-five minutes to explain some of what he has been researching. He has also spent a good deal of his latest research on that portion of the plates entrusted to Joseph Smith that were sealed. What do we know about the sealed parts? And if you listen carefully, you will learn from Sam here what that portion of the plates is called." Bender displayed his golden smile. It had all the warmth of a dear friend as he introduced Samuel. "I won't steal your thunder, Sam. You step over here, and I'll sit in your place while you address this rather informed group of scholars. If anyone in the dining room should find your information interesting, I hope you don't mind them eavesdropping."

"Not at all, Sid," Samuel replied, rising from his chair.

* * *

He trotted along the sidewalk hugging the bushes, silently slid through the door Roy had carelessly left unlocked, and stepped into the foyer of the Book of Mormon Center. The regulation exit lights cast an eerie glow over the area, providing enough light for Jeremiah to make his way to the far side of the building. The path around the arena was covered in green carpeting. It muted any sound Jeremiah would otherwise have made groping along the hall to the section where a light glowed beyond an open door. He could hear Roy punching numbers on the telephone. He had already booted up his computer and was calling someone. It didn't matter. He had his skinny back to the door, so he didn't see Jeremiah as he silently edged into the room filled with sound equipment. One wall was lined with tapes, CDs, and books. On the other was a long console, the type that any self-respecting recording studio would have. A mike stood dead center. Jeremiah eased around the equipment, staying well out of Roy's line of peripheral vision.

As he listened to Meyers' answering machine, Roy must have heard the faint rustle of the Albertsons shopping bags as Jeremiah removed them from his sleeve. He started to turn around when Jeremiah sprang into action. Gripping the bags in both hands, he brought them down firmly over Roy's head and pulled them tightly around his neck.

With a shocked reflex, Roy tried to lift himself out of his swivel desk chair in violent protest. His mouth gaped open, his eyes widened as he gasped for air. The plastic was plastered to Roy's lips as he struggled for air that wasn't available. He fell backwards into Jeremiah's chest, the back of his head striking Jeremiah's upper arm. In one giant movement, Jeremiah kicked Roy's feet out in front of him and he fell back hard into the chair. His right foot crashed into the monitor on the desk, shattering the glass. He tried again, only to have his feet slip and cause him to grab for any object within his grasp. He fought hard, but Jeremiah was a powerful man. After several minutes of struggle, Roy's limp body collapsed.

Jeremiah let Roy's body drop to the floor. Then he reached up in the paneling of the lowered ceiling and ripped out the smoke alarm wiring; with his lighter he set the plastic covering of the console on fire. It took a moment to spread.

The only sound to be heard was the crackling of the spreading flames. They rapidly spread from the false ceiling and engulfed the sound panel and other equipment in the room as Jeremiah moved back and watched the fire consume everything in its path. The kid's body would be charred in minutes. Now the flames encircled the room where Jeremiah stood a moment longer, convinced the destruction would be total.

He knew the autopsy report on Roy would read: "Death due to deprivation of oxygen." So they wouldn't find smoke in the lungs. What difference would that make? Provo, Jeremiah was convinced, would not have the forensic specialists of a city like Los Angeles or New York. No way. They might get an expert from Salt Lake City. So what? He would be long gone. He knew how to cover his tracks. He took pride in his destructive work. After all, he was considered in his circle one of the best—a real pro. In seconds he would be dashing for his pickup, and soon thereafter on the road back to Wyoming and the shelter of the compound. The Oracle would be pleased with his work. He was certain of that.

* * *

Samuel stood at the head of the table shaking his head, saying he didn't mind if Bender stole a little thunder. As he stood he wished that Dr. Polk and Stephen had come with him, but Polk was weak and unable to attend. And Stephen had his own set of concerns to attend to. He would do it alone.

"I'll go right to the presentation of what we have uncovered thus far in our research. It is moving along very well, as you will see."

Samuel's grandson, Brad, had no time for food. He would grab a bite later. He had made three trips back and forth to the Center's van for equipment. He had set up the monitor for the video and laid out notes on a small table a waiter had supplied for him.

"My grandson Brad has been of great assistance on our journey to gather information. If you will turn your attention to the screen," invited Samuel as he nodded to the waiter who quickly stepped to a panel of light switches on the far wall and doused all the overhead lights in half of the dining room. Most of the patrons preferred candlelight to bright lights, so it hardly made a difference when part of the large room went shadowy with flickering candlelight.

Samuel began with confidence and notes. For the next several minutes he covered everything from the restoration of the gospel to the conversion of the Jews as he moved quickly through the chronology of events to the present. The most startling information he dispensed by way of film and lecture was the return of the remnant of Jacob. It got a response when Harry Child asked if Samuel really believed that a part of the Nephites survived and would return as the remnant of Jacob. All listened intently. Among the group were those who thought differently. It nearly lead to a debate, but Samuel avoided dwelling on the subject and quickly moved to the gathering of the House of Israel, of which the last to be gathered would be the Jews. Brad had a good amount of footage from the Holy Land to project for the enjoyment of the group, the most vital of which was Morris Herschner's announcement about Solomon's Temple site. It was not where the Dome of the Rock was blocking it as everyone had supposed. Fantastic news. Now the Jews had their own open space to build on.

* * *

The task of carrying in moving boxes had hung over Stephen's head for the past week. Now he struggled with a heavier-than-normal box he had brought into the house from the garage. It was big, too big to be lugging when he was this tired. He steadied the box against the kitchen door frame while he reached in and clicked on the outside light so he would not stumble on the step up. He was still not too familiar with the new house. As he entered, the phone in the kitchen rang. He set the box down inside the back door while the phone rang a second time.

Stephen grabbed the receiver and pulled it to his ear after the third ring. Out of breath from his exertion, he puffed out the words, "Stephen Thorn."

It was Todd. "Dad! You won't believe what's happening!" Todd yelled into the phone, panic in his voice.

"What?" Stephen shouted.

"The Center's on fire. Get down here! I mean it's going up in flames; there must be five fire engines here trying to put it out. Dad, get down here. Max and I saw the flames while we were driving by. We stopped at Burger King after class and were on our way home to see a couple of friends."

"Where are you now?"

"I'm at a pay phone down the street, but I can still see the flames shooting up from here. I don't believe what's happening."

"I'm coming!" Stephen slammed the phone on its hook and shouted for Anney to hurry. "There's a fire at the Center!"

\* \* \*

Fred Himmer was the first to ask Samuel a question after Samuel explained that the world was moving rapidly toward fulfillment of one of the major prophetic happenings in the last days. Samuel yielded the floor to Himmer. Letting the group pop questions was a method Samuel had employed as a mission president in Japan. It generally set a more casual mood if the questions were not barbed.

Himmer's long, drawn features stood out in relief against very white skin and ice-blue eyes that seemed to look deeply into Samuel's. He felt a twinge of resentment come over him as Fred Himmer, a scholar's scholar who no longer taught in the Church Education program but spent much of his years in retirement working over prophecy, had written a book in the early 1970s that refuted much of the then-current thinking on events of the Church and the world as they awaited the Savior. He took little stock in what the early members of the Twelve had to say about the Rocky Mountain Saints leading out in the return to Jackson County to build the New Jerusalem and the temple. The book had been poorly received by all but those few who agreed that much of the prophecy in the *Journal of Discourses* by men such as the Pratt brothers and others on what they thought they heard the Prophet Joseph Smith say about the Saints' return to Jackson County was suspect.

In his comments, Himmer had been quick to point out that much of what the early leaders said on the subject was what someone else said that the Prophet Joseph had said. Even the "yellow dog" statement attributed to Brigham Young was secondhand. It was a "someone said he said . . . " All of this Himmer had attributed to third-party hearsay accounts. He had been quick to point out that it was not good scholarship. And even more to the point, it likely was in error.

Himmer trudged on about his research into hearsay in Mormonism as Samuel stood waiting to continue. He respected Himmer, but the man was taking far more time to make his point than needed, which was not a question but sheer grandstanding. Himmer pounded on. "I thank you for listening to an old man, and I would like to rehearse some of my findings on the subject of the return of the Ten Tribes and what we know of their return." Himmer wiped his thin lips that had saliva forming at the corners. He made a long pause, then said, "Brother Meyers, many of the details are missing, but we do know they will return as a body out of the north country. From where they will come, we haven't yet been told. As all of you know, the Ten Tribes of Israel were taken captive by the Assyrians, located about 500 miles north of Israel. The location may be present-day Turkey. They were held captive for a little less than a hundred years. The tribes escaped from their captors and what we know of their escape is found in apocryphal writings. Esdras tells us the Ten Tribes went forth 'unto a further country where never man dwelt. That they might there keep their statutes, which they never kept in their own land.'"

Samuel and the others knew these facts, yet they tolerated Himmer's rehearsed presentation of the facts.

"I accept that," Himmer said, seeming to be oblivious to the group's desire to move along with Samuel's presentation. "I think they repented of much of their heathen ways, and with this reformed attitude the Ten Tribes went deep into the north. Some of our Church leaders have said the Ten Tribes, as they moved north, were led by prophets and inspired leaders. We learned from the Prophet Joseph that later, in the course of their history, John the Revelator was among them. Where are they now? This has been a topic of discussion without resolution for over a hundred years. The Church has an official position on this. In brief, they tell us that no one knows. Not a few of the early Church leaders stated that the Ten Tribes were whisked away from the earth, that they now reside on a planet somewhere in the universe. Orson Pratt claimed he heard the Prophet Joseph say the Ten Tribes were broken off much like the City of Enoch, and that in the last days they will be brought back and let down in the polar region. Brigham Young, according to Wilford Woodruff, felt the Ten Tribes were on a portion of earth separated from the main body."

Shaking his thin head, Himmer said, "Where they are is not the issue. It's their glorious return I have focused on. I believe the return of the Lost Ten Tribes will be a unique, specific, physical happening. There is far too much scriptural evidence to refute that statement. I'll spare you many of the details." That statement alone pleased the group. "Still, I'll say this much: Jeremiah tells us the return will be so miraculous an event that other events of the time will pale, and it will be far greater than when the Lord led Israel out of Egypt.

"What's more," Himmer raised his voice, "look for a large body to come down from the ice lands. It was Nephi who said, 'Yea, the more part of all the tribes have been led away.' Take a look at the Doctrine and Covenants, section 133. Here you find the most detailed discussion of the actual return. This scripture tells us they will strike the ice and a highway will be cast up in the midst of the great deep. It says a lot more about their coming, but we all know from revelation that they will bring their record with them. I find this appealing. They will come with their prophets, the priesthood; and John the Revelator will be with them. They will come to the City of Zion and there receive their endowments. They will remain only a while in the New Jerusalem; then, following the great battle of Armageddon, they will go to Palestine to fulfill prophecy that says they will return to their homeland and there join with their brethren, the tribe of Judah."

Himmer looked about him. He removed his white, starched handkerchief and wiped more saliva from the corners of his mouth. Samuel had the uncomfortable impression that he was just getting started. He did what he was forced to do. He cut Himmer off with one comment. "However, Brother Himmer, you perhaps are right on several points, but the coming of the Ten Tribes is not the key issue in the coming of the Savior. That will come later in the chronology of events. A significant event has to happen first before we get to that stage in our preparation for the Second Coming. We have misread this key event, or rather ignored it altogether in our discussions in the Church. Because we have done so, the whole Church is under condemnation."

Himmer said with a shade of realization that he had taken Samuel's time and ought not to have. "I'm just trying to be thought provoking. Sorry I took so much of your time, Samuel."

"You are thought provoking, I'll grant you that. In fact, you have caused me to remember a little known prophecy by Nephi, that the Nephites would obtain the very scriptures of the Lost Tribes. When? In the future."

"First, let me remind you we are the Gentiles who are to receive the book spoken of by Nephi in 2 Nephi 30:3. This is a vital concept to comprehend. If you follow the course of events in the last days Nephi has made it abundantly clear in I Nephi 13:42 that the gospel will be taken to the Gentiles first—us. We are those Gentiles who have received the gospel in this day."

At the far side of the table a dainty hand went up. Karen Zuker from the religion department at Brigham Young University wanted to ask a question. "Brother Meyers, are you saying that those of us in the Church are Gentiles? I'm of the impression that once we join the Church, we are no longer Gentiles but of the House of Israel. Have I been wrong all these years?"

Samuel moved a step to his right to be more in direct line with the petite questioner. "As Church members we have indeed been adopted into the House of Israel, but that does not affect our national citizenship. Patriarchal blessings do not change our nationality. Nephi told us the Book of Mormon would go to the Gentiles in the last days and be carried to the world by them, particularly to the remnant of Jacob."

"But my patriarchal blessing states I am of the lineage of Ephraim. I'm sure most of us in this room are from Ephraim. Ephraim was the son of Joseph, who was of the House of Israel. Am I wrong?"

"No. You have been fully adopted into the House of Israel and designated as part of the lineage of Ephraim. In fact, you may have some of the blood of Ephraim in your ancestry. I'm sure many of us do. What we really are I call *covenant Gentiles*."

# Chapter 8

Jeremiah was too experienced to take a direct route out of Provo to Salt Lake City. As he veered to the right and started into Provo Canyon, he had that exquisite sensation, erotic in its intensity, of having taken what he thought of as a worthless life. Only he could savor this moment in its sheer joy. He would not even let the Oracle in on the joy he now felt. It was too personal for anyone but himself to know its depth. For him there was no greater worldly pleasure than knowing he could take another person's life—snuff it without regard for foolish man-made laws.

\* \* \*

"Are you Mr. Meyers, sir?" the waiter asked in a smooth, quiet, upbeat tone of voice next to Samuel who had turned to face the young man who had tapped him on the shoulder.

Samuel leaned his ear toward the voice. "Yes, I am."

"I'm sorry to interrupt you, but you have an urgent call, sir. You can take it at the receptionist's desk if you like."

Samuel's heart skipped. Urgency meant emergency; emergency meant that something happened that would perhaps be troubling—family? What? He excused himself and followed the waiter toward the reception desk. It was Stephen who in a hurried voice told Samuel that the Center was going up in flames. "Get down here as fast as you can. I don't believe what is happening. It just can't be happening. Todd says the whole thing's going up in flames. Hurry!"

Samuel quickly returned to the group and explained that he and Brad would have to leave immediately. Then he told them that a fire was raging out of control at the Book of Mormon Center in Provo.

\* \* \*

Todd and Max paid no attention to the cops directing traffic at the intersection as residents from nearby apartments and homes raced up the center of Canyon Drive to get a view of the flaming Center. The fire was too intense for any man to run up the south side of the street. When they were half a block from the crumbling building, they stood transfixed, staring in shock. The black smoke continued to pour out of the building and climb like puffs of angry clouds to the heavens. It was the worst smoke pollution Provo had endured in months.

Todd and Max dared not get closer. They stood in the street, unable to do anything to salvage things in the Center. They felt as if they were watching a video of Sherman's burning of Atlanta depicted in *Gone with the Wind* as the roof caved in with a crash. It was so unbelievable, so terrible. Did Roy leave some electrical thing on? Did something go berserk that should have been switched off? As the two college students stood in the middle of the street, a five-inch fire hose slid like a python up against their shoes as the firemen worked the flames twenty feet in front of them. They knew they were in the wrong place, but they had a right to be here. "This can't be happening," Todd kept mumbling. "It simply can't be."

It was Max who asked the heart-wrenching question of Todd, "Isn't that Roy's van parked over there?"

"Where?" Todd asked urgently.

"Over there at the front of the building. Do you see it?"

"Yeah," Todd breathed. "It's his."

Todd stared at Max, heartsick at seeing the singed vehicle he was certain was Roy's.

"Isn't Roy somewhere in Wyoming tonight?" Max asked, as concerned as Todd for the welfare of their friend.

"I don't know, I hope so. But if I recall, he was returning this evening. Naw. He must have left his van parked there while he is gone."

"No, they don't park cars that close to the entrance during the day. Tourist busses have to unload."

Max paused, turning wide eyes to Todd whose reaction was the same: "Do you think Roy was in the building? Do you think the firemen know that someone might have been in the Center this evening?"

Todd shook his head over and over, mumbling, "This is incredible. It isn't happening."

Max was stunned, too. Roy was such a great guy. The two of them had liked each other when they first met through Dr. Polk and Stephen. They had a lot in common—both sort of loners and both into computers. Roy had taught Max some hi-tech tricks he could never have learned on his own. He desperately hoped Roy was not in the Center. An uneasy feeling was growing inside Max's mind. He knew Roy had gone to Gateway this weekend . . . There couldn't possibly be a connection between Roy's tour and this fire, could there?

# Chapter 9

"Dad, Mom! Over here!" Todd started running toward a police car just pulling into the parking lot, waving for his dad to follow. Todd shouted his concerns, trying to be heard over the hiss of water hitting the front end of Roy's burning van, that Roy might be inside the building. When he saw Roy's flame-endangered car in front of the Center, Stephen, too, felt terrified that Roy had returned and was inside the building when the fire broke out. It made sense. But how could anyone enter that inferno now? More importantly, how could Roy possibly survive? Stephen knew he couldn't, and so did Todd. It was too horrible to comprehend as the boy ran toward his father in desperation. Stephen calmed Todd by suggesting that Roy's van must be moved away from the fire. They asked the fire chief to move it. It was one small, positive thing they could concentrate on at this moment of sheer destruction.

\* \* \*

Reuben seldom left Gateway. He always felt more secure once he closed the eight-foot gate behind him inside the sprawling compound in the craggy mountains. Gateway's full compound was hidden beyond the ridge, but the gated, state-of-the-art community began its tightly guarded security at the gate that faced north onto ranch lands.

Reuben had been chief of security at the compound for five years. In reality, Gateway had only been a dream of the Oracle five years ago. Nevertheless, the Oracle had Reuben in place while construction on the dream ensued in the mountains. It had been his job to secure the fencing surrounding the two thousand-acre layout. The Oracle insisted their meeting had been the will of God. Reuben was hired one rainy night as a temp by the Beagle Security Agency in Seattle to help guard a Mr. Alexander Josiah DeWitt, millionaire plus, who was selling his stock to raise funds to build his new Utopian dream city.

There had been well-to-do, interested parties in Seattle who had come to listen to Josiah tell of his dream and the need for converts. Security was tight the evening Reuben first saw the Oracle. Someone earlier in the day had called the police to inform them he hated all the Oracle stood for and was going to kill him. He didn't explain how, but the Oracle's front men wanted extra guards on hand at the Clarion Hotel where the Oracle would be speaking at a dinner of carefully selected guests.

Reuben had arrived early for security detail, and after one of the Oracle's staff members checked his background, he asked that Reuben stand at the door to the Oracle's suite and remain there all evening to ensure that no unauthorized person entered the suite. Everyone needed clearance. It was an easy assignment for Reuben.

It wasn't until the evening was over that Reuben met the Oracle Josiah. With three staff members trailing, the Oracle stepped off the elevator on the top floor and moved with a determined stride to the door of his suite. Reuben bowed slightly toward the Oracle, then with immense charm the Oracle extended his hand to Reuben, introduced himself, and thanked him for his service that evening.

"What is your name?" the Oracle had asked. At that moment Reuben recalled his initial meeting with the perceptive Oracle and explaining that he was available and clever. The Oracle had hired him on the spot to travel with him on his next conversion tour, which would last three months. Reuben had no family or ties to keep him in Seattle. As a matter of fact, he had already made up his mind to leave and move to Las Vegas where security work for a man with his experience paid a fair salary.

A month into the tour, Reuben was promoted to head of the Oracle's traveling security force. At the end of the tour, Reuben stayed on to set up an elaborate system to guard the future Gateway project. His role was established and his job secure. What the Oracle sensed in Reuben was the hungry look of a human predator, a man with no soul who could carry out harsh commands in the interest of maintaining order and security. Reuben knew his business well. He had trained in Army Special Forces; he once took an assignment with a deranged heart surgeon who bought an island off the coast of Central America and trained mercenaries for hire. Reuben concealed that two-year episode in his training from all but the Oracle. Recognizing his own kind, Reuben spoke of the experience in some detail when the Oracle interviewed him for the position of chief of security.

Unknown to Reuben, the Oracle was already aware of Reuben's extensive exploits as a mercenary. He frankly told Reuben he admired a man of action, one not hesitant to carry out orders, any orders—even executions. Reuben was well suited to implement the security tasks in his charge. Roy's elimination last night had been one of several he had orchestrated over the past five years. It was simply part of his job description—all designed to keep order at Gateway. Whatever had to be done was done without feeling or remorse. It was primarily the iron will Reuben displayed that pleased the Oracle most and caused him to lavish gifts and special favors on his chief of security.

Even now, as Reuben reported on the success of the ordered execution, he offered the grisly details in a professional manner, a touch of pride in his voice. The Oracle listened to the particulars without comment while he dried his still firm body with a large, white towel. He had enjoyed his morning swim in his indoor pool on the south wing of the main compound. Always concerned about his health, he had the pool cleaned and filled each week with spring water brought in by a tanker truck.

"So, you took care of our little matter?"

"Yes, sir. There is not a trace of evidence that it was anything but an accident. Jeremiah used what he calls his snuff method to execute Roy, and with the intense heat and flames his body was charred almost beyond recognition. I heard a news report on KSL this morning that the body was found inside the gutted Center. The news indicated that it appeared to be an accident."

"Well done," the Oracle praised, watching Reuben's face carefully. "I would like you to send someone into Jackson this morning to pick up a new Jeep Cherokee I ordered with all the bells and whistles. It is your present from me for a job well done. Thank you, Reuben."

Reuben's beaming face told Josiah all he needed to know. The gift of the Cherokee would mask any hint that the Oracle was displeased with his security chief. He would never suspect anything to the contrary.

And Reuben didn't. Working for the Oracle wasn't half bad. Reuben ignored the many other traits about him that would have troubled a less experienced man. He liked having the full backing of a crazy man imbued with religion.

# Chapter 10

They sat across from one another. Samuel leaned back on the sofa in his small apartment, while Bender leaned forward in an overstuffed chair to the right. Samuel had woven his fingers into a cup and with elbows pointed out on the sides he held the back of his head by his laced fingers. It was his method of relaxation, though at the moment his mind was too riveted on the tragedy at the Book of Mormon Center two nights ago and the loss of Roy Carver to focus on the subject Bender had come to discuss.

Right now he wanted a breather from the stresses of the day. On the other hand, Samuel admitted to himself, maybe by talking about something, anything but the horrors of the fire, he could escape the oppression he had experienced for the past thirty-six hours. Talk of the fire was everywhere on the street. Those who knew that Samuel had a connection to the Center offered their regrets and mentioned to him what a loss it was.

Samuel decided to make the most of this session with Bender. It could not go longer than an hour, but he would give him that much time. He was to rejoin Katherine, who was at the Thorns', and work through the sorrow by taking a long walk along the river footpath before dark.

Sidney's eagerness to listen and learn about the events of the Second Coming were uppermost in his mind. For one thing, he hadn't known Roy, and Samuel had to admit that he, too, had not been that deeply involved with the young man. Roy had been part of the team, but he and Samuel had gone off in separate directions and reported back to Peter Polk periodically. It wasn't as if Samuel had lost a member of his family. A friend, yes; someone he admired, of course. But the association ended there. Why shouldn't they discuss the coming events that Sidney had come over to learn about? Samuel had invited him to his apartment before leaving Jerusalem. "Why don't you come to my apartment on the Friday after the lecture?" he had said before Bender left with his tour. Samuel had failed to cancel the appointment; with all that had happened, it had completely slipped his mind. He happened to be at his apartment picking up a

91

heavy jacket for the walk with Katherine when the doorbell sounded. Rather than disappoint Sid, even though he had every reason to not spend time with him since there was so much sadness, he decided to take a moment and follow up on their appointment.

"You mentioned all of this gathering, Sam. But unless I missed something, you didn't mention anything about your great find on the coming events. I know you think I'm a pest on this issue, but you did promise to let me in on it. So . . . I'm waiting."

"I know you are, but let's take a step at a time, okay? Let's talk about the gathering first."

"Okay, but I do want to know what you seem to have found out that is so startling. I am confused about the gathering. I don't know whether you are talking about the members of Church, Lost Tribes, the Lamanites, or the House of Israel. I have a pretty good idea; however, I need clarification."

"Okay. First, though, let's back up. We have already talked about the Times of the Gentiles. As I see it, the Times of the Gentiles will conclude about the time the remnant of Jacob will return, and we will have real internal strife at that time. The major nations of the earth will be struggling financially and politically."

"How soon do you expect this to happen?" asked Bender.

"I don't know the exact time. I think it's close, but I don't really know. I do think that the cause will be destructive forces all over the world. Mostly politically motivated conflict, making it unsafe for our missionaries to continue proselyting."

"What exactly do you mean by destruction? It is too soon in the sequence of events for the terrible destruction of Armageddon to explode. Don't you agree?"

"No doubt. Armageddon, as I see it, will happen later. There has to be the gathering of the House of Israel before that last great and terrible battle. However, I'm talking about the whole earth being in commotion, governments failing, civil war—perhaps even war in our own land. Throughout the world there will be disruption of commerce, communications, armies on the move, leaders going off the deep end. The wicked shall slay the wicked, and fear shall come upon every man."

"Yes, that's scriptural."

"It seems to me that corruption and vice will be at an all-time high and people will revolt. This of course is not the end, by which I mean the ushering in of the Millennial Reign. There is still a long haul after the Times of the Gentiles is fulfilled. It may appear to be the end and many will think of it as the windup, but for the righteous Saints and the remnant of Jacob whom the Lord has foretold will return to this land, it will be seen as a time of cleansing and a new beginning. I'm certain the living prophet will give direction to the members. What a time we're going to have when whole cities are left devoid of people so that the remnant of Jacob can be housed, or as Isaiah said, 'inherit the Gentiles and make the desolate cities to be inhabited.' It will certainly be a shaking down of corruption and cleansing the country. The loose-willed and the immoral will be either destroyed or cast out. It will also be a time, I'm sure, when the missionaries come home."

"By home, what do you think this means? Where is home?"

"Good question. For the most part I think it is wherever Zion is well established. It could be anywhere in the world: Europe, Asia, South America, all these locations. You know Africa is a growing area of the Church. Home for the African is Africa. Home for the Saints, as I see it, is wherever the stakes of Zion are located."

"Yeah, I'm aware of that. But isn't it interesting you would say Africa? Back when Crowther was writing his book, he showed graphically how the Saints would gather to the mountains and go as a body to build the New Jerusalem. Now, the Church is so far flung one wonders how that would be possible."

"That could happen, but I doubt it. I can't read into what the Savior has told us in the Book of Mormon that the gathering of the Saints will be to one place. It may be that we will meet in the mountains, but I doubt it. As a body the Church is becoming too large. Can you imagine pulling twelve million or more members into the Salt Lake Valley in one giant roundup of Saints to head to Missouri? Besides, such a theory lacks scriptural backing. The stakes of Zion are the gathering points and the protective shield for the Saints right wherever they happen to be located. To me it makes more sense. Even if it's downtown New York that they gather, and stand in holy places, and not be moved, they will be blessed by remaining in the stakes of Zion. That means almost everywhere in the world."

"I have to agree with you, Sam. As I see it, at the rate we are building temples, there may be temples dotting the land when the Times of the Gentiles is finished. Temples will be everywhere, and I doubt that the Lord is going to abandon all those temples. Wherever the saints are called to stand, I suppose that is what is meant by 'called home,' and righteous homes, chapels, and temples are holy places."

"Sure. In the case of the missionaries of North America, it will be here in the United States. Some of the early thinkers on this matter, back in the time of Brigham Young, naturally thought of the security of the Rockies. They may not have had in mind the growth and flooding of the earth with righteousness and truth to gather out God's elect from the four quarters of the earth, as foretold in the Book of Moses, which Joseph Smith said would be done by men and angels. This, I am certain, will be after the New Jerusalem is built and the Zion of Enoch returns, whose angelic inhabitants can labor with righteous men to flood the earth with the gospel."

"Wait, I'm still learning. Of course I've studied the phases, but I've never taught or had deep discussions on the things that are to come. I'm just a babe in the woods, Sam," Bender pleaded.

"Not hardly. Not you. You must have a working knowledge of what is to come. All you need is a little more clarification."

"In your research, you have certainly shown me that you already know more about the events of the Second Coming, I would venture to guess, than nearly anyone in the Church." Bender pointed his finger at Samuel and followed it with his comments. "For years I somehow had in my mind the traditional view that the Saints would trek back to Missouri and build the city of Zion, and somehow everything would be peaceful and secure."

"For a segment of worthy Saints that may be true. Nothing tells us that all the Saints will go to Jackson County. It is too small to hold all the members, even now, at least in a conventional living arrangement of agriculture and industry. No, there will be those who will help build the city and remain to inhabit it, but it seems to me that either the city will rapidly expand and all the Saints will find a home there eventually, or the Saints will continue to live in their own regions of the world and teach the gospel to those who will make up the second phase of the gathering."

"And that second phase includes?"

"We'll get to that in a moment. When the New Jerusalem is constructed and functioning and expanding, then the gathering of all Israel will commence, beginning with the Lamanites."

"I've read where the city of the New Jerusalem will, in time, cover all of North and South America. That's a big city."

"But think who'll be there—there will be the remnant of Jacob, the Covenant Gentiles; the City of Enoch will return to its former location, and the Ten Tribes and the Jews will be in their own land. That is the order scheduled by the Lord. When the tiny little body of Saints who made up the Church April 6, 1830, gathered to officially restore the Church, they started this mighty gathering process. What an ambitious group they were to think they were at the head of the greatest missionary work to ever take place. You know, sometimes I think we lose sight of that goal because we aren't aware that all Israel will be gathered into the gospel net after the New Jerusalem is built."

Samuel's phone rang. He abruptly interrupted the conversation and grabbed it. Katherine was calling. "Sam, I really have to get out of here for a spell. Your Dr. Polk has come by with his male nurse. There is so much weeping and great sorrow. If you can, why don't you come and get me. Okay?"

"I'll be right there."

He placed the phone back on the cradle and mentioned to Bender that he had to leave. "I know we didn't get too far, but I have to drive over and pick up Katherine. Things are pretty sad over there."

Bender got to his feet and nodded agreement. "Sure, Sam. You need to go."

"Oh, one other thing before we get out of here. I'm going out to visit with a young man you might be interested to meet, if you have time tomorrow afternoon. I set up the appointment this morning and told him I might bring a friend."

"What's he doing that you think I would be interested to know?"

"He's been a real support of the Center, an admirer of Peter Polk."

"Who is he?"

"Dunfee, the fellow who built that big computer hardware company—you know, the one west of Alpine. I heard where he's involved with some high-tech communication that ties in with eventual disruption of the social and economic order of things. He really believes our country will experience great turmoil. I have to agree. He is the one I'm taking you to meet. We have a two o'clock appointment. I'll pick you up."

"How did you hear about what he's up to?"

"He's very interested in our Book of Mormon Center. I think he will help us get back on our feet. He has already offered a piece of property at his large complex near Alpine. We have turned it down. It's too far from the freeway and any easy access by tourists."

* * *

The letter was brief, but cheerful. How could Anney know that it was a forgery of Brenda's handwriting? She accepted the shape of the letters, the tone of the phrases as those of her lovely daughter. She would not have any suspicion that the words were anything but Brenda's. To the extent that she heard from Brenda, Anney was pleased. That she hadn't divulged her whereabouts depressed Anney. She read it with red eyes, more because of the sad news about Roy than the fact that Brenda remained at a secret location.

She had wept most of the morning at the tragedy of Roy's death. When Katherine came over, the two rehashed over the kitchen table what they had heard about the fire. When the mail arrived, Katherine was just leaving, having offered all the solace she could muster. She had assured Anney that death was a constant in her life. She had lost two husbands, made adjustments in life, and assured Anney that life would go on. Of course there is a mourning period, but that too passes, she had told Anney.

After Anney saw Katherine depart for a walk with Samuel, she went to the mailbox at the curb. Stephen had erected a black box with white lettering the week before. She had emptied it the day before when it was stuffed with bills, notices, and junk mail. Today as she peeked inside she saw only one letter. She recognized the envelope and handwriting: Brenda had sent a letter. In spite of the glumness of the day, Anney was excited to hear from her daughter. She stood next to the mailbox and ripped off the top of the envelope to get at the news.

*Dearest Dad & Mom,*

*I'm still not at liberty to divulge my location, but I should be calling you soon, maybe. I just hate not letting you know exactly where I am and what I'm*

*doing, but it is part of the order to remain silent in these matters. Understand?*
*I will not be writing you for a couple of weeks. The director told us that we*
*need to spend more time in meditation than writing home. I'm not sure I agree.*
*It is therapeutic for me to write to you.*

*I'm learning so many worthwhile things about the spirit of man and how*
*we can all reach our inner selves through certain exercises. It is too lengthy to*
*explain, but maybe in my next letter I will.*

*I do love you and Todd so much.*

*Love, Brenda*

Anney felt relieved that Brenda sounded so cheerful. Each letter came with
such hope and promise. Anney stared across the asphalt road to the place under
construction across the street. It would be twice as large as her house but,
Anney consoled herself, not nearly so homey. She was about to step back from
the mailbox when it struck her that most of Brenda's letters said the same thing.
She wondered why. Brenda was a talker. Most of her early letters from college
were filled with details about campus life and the boys she was meeting. These
letters from somewhere were void of Brenda's talent for gushy details. Totally
unlike her.

* * *

Jeremiah was at the computer by late morning. The trip back from Provo
a couple nights ago had consumed much of that night. He had carefully stayed
well within the posted speed limits. He slouched sideways, his feet propped up,
his tooled cowboy boots digging into the chair next to him. He had been surfing
the net for half an hour when Martha entered the compound's nerve center.
Both security men were off checking a malfunctioning monitor. They trusted
Jeremiah to hold down the fort, something he did very well. The events of the
night before had left him drowsy, but after four hours of rest, he was up and at
it. Of all the locations in the compound, it was the communications structure
which housed the electronic equipment that gave Jeremiah recreation, a sense
of community with the world, and a totally secret hideaway within the
compound that protected him from snoops in the form of federal officials.

He sat with his eyes intensely focused on the computer's monitor. He loved
exploring various Web sites. He knew it was his escape from his surroundings.
His confinement to the cave was beginning to wear on his nerves. He had been

outside the complex but four times in two years. His venture as far as Provo had seemed to him like an outing. The business he took care of in Provo had only added to the excitement of future jobs.

*The men I knew in prison have it easier than I do in some ways. But I'm getting out. One more hit, one more poor sucker like that Roy, just one more at $30,000 a hit, and I'll have the money I set out to stash away. One more,* he reasoned as he sat bored with the chat group he had tied into. *Those guys at least get a yard break out in the sunshine.* Jeremiah seldom left the cave, and when he did, it was at night. Members of Gateway security knew who he was, but few of the youthful members of the compound would recognize him. That was okay. He had a fetish for keeping a low profile. The Internet, with all of its variety of weirdos and misfits on the dozens of chat groups, kept his thoughts alive. He especially liked a couple of the chat groups that debated the dynamics of murder and ways to conceal it. He observed some brilliant minds discuss the pros and cons of bombings, while other chat groups debated the best way to remove a life through a variety of instruments. He had little patience for those who posted their stupid comments on the screen. They were totally inexperienced in the art of killing! Jeremiah knew. He was a pro.

He thought how inept some of the interlopers in the chat group were. He had been on line nearly two years and by now had acquired some information and finesse on the World Wide Web. He could tell those with experience from those with none. He always perked up when those he considered pros came on line, but they were rare. Most, he decided, knew nothing about killing. He didn't buy the idea that law enforcement officials of developed nations observed the treaty that they not monitor chat groups. He sensed that no law enforcement agency would pass up the opportunity to spy, since the on-line groups were so accessible. He wondered how professional one could be as an assassin to get on the Net and discuss it openly, but some did. He wouldn't. He prided himself on his ability to remain in the shadows. Still, there were times when Jeremiah was convinced he was reading the words of a pro. Regardless of the amateurish nature of the chat groups, Jeremiah found them a diversion.

The professional hit man didn't see Martha slip into the room. He sat with his back to the main entrance of the command/communications center. The hood of his Gap sweatshirt drooped behind his shaved head. He looked for all the world like a monk at meditation. From time to time he glanced at the monitors that electronically recorded movements throughout the compound, from the twelve-foot-high fence on the east, to the rock wall on the west, and all the buildings and paths in-between. It was an elaborate system of checks on the movements of people. Jeremiah had the ability to spot action like a master air controller. He could monitor eight screens at once and still fool with the Net.

"I don't know how you do it," Martha said quietly as she moved in beside Jeremiah. She looked like everybody's uptight aunt: bone thin, firm jaw, never quick to smile.

Her voice that shattered the stillness in the command center would have startled any normal person. Not Jeremiah. He had felt her presence behind his back seconds before she spoke. His talent for detection and surveillance had not been learned. Like a Burmese tiger, it was genetic.

He said nothing for at least a minute, continuing to follow the conversation between the imbeciles on the Net. Satisfied that they were amateurs at taking life, he punched the power button under the screen, causing a sudden green-and-white flash of light to streak across the screen before it went dark. Jeremiah turned in the swivel desk chair to lock onto Martha's light green eyes, eyes that revealed nothing. He knew her type. She had the New York City smarts of the woman she was plus the cunning of a cobra. Jeremiah knew they were a pair. The attraction they felt for one another was purely business. Each knew that the Oracle needed their particular talents for control, and each knew that the other was highly professional. There was nothing in human nature that they hadn't seen to one degree or another. They had the instincts of terrorists and the ability to manage lives—snuff them out if it came to that. There seemed to be no surface sentimentality or easy access to either of them. It was a mutual admiration of evil that tied them together and cemented their relationship. For a couple of months now, the two had been meeting sporadically to converse in an easy manner, though warily still. Martha had come in for such a brief session.

Their conversation drifted from one topic to another. At one point Martha wanted to know the great attraction the Net held for Jeremiah. He shrugged. "It's harmless. I can travel the world in all these sites and pop in on any stupid conversation I want with the click of a mouse. And you know what? I can feel superior to the idiots out there who write endlessly about things they know nothing about."

"You like to feel superior?"

"Don't you?"

"I don't know. I don't know what I like anymore." The inflection in Martha's voice was mellow and softer than Jeremiah had heard before.

"Come on, Mother Martha, you're not going to unload on me today? One thing I admire about you is your sense of detachment to things emotional. Don't get soft on me."

"You know, I do have feelings."

"No, I didn't know. I thought you had seared those long ago. You're in the wrong work to start getting sentimental at this stage. The Oracle hired you, as he did me, because of your steel nerves and complete detachment from anything around you. Perk up," he said with a lilt in his voice. "This is not you. At least not the Martha I know."

"It's not always easy for me to be what you call detached. I wonder sometimes just what I'm doing in this compound. 'Why do I do what I do?' I ask myself."

"Let me put your troubled mind at ease." Jeremiah reached over and tapped Martha's loose, cotton, flowered dress at the knee. She withdrew the knee slightly. He had never touched her before. Jeremiah sensed her reserve. He didn't care. He had touched other women. They meant nothing to him, including this one—no attachment. "You're doing it for the same reason that I do what I'm hired to do: You do it for the money. We both know that when we've socked away a tidy sum, we'll retire from this scene."

"Do you really think the Oracle will let us just walk out the front gate when we think we've had enough?"

"No, but think ahead; don't walk out the front gate. There will be ways to exit. But we're not ready for that step yet, are we? At least I'm not ready. My little nest egg is still building in my numbered account in the Caymans." Jeremiah took his unblinking eyes from their locked gaze on Martha to look up and study the surveillance monitors.

No unusual action.

He turned back to her green eyes. "You know, Martha, you are something of an expert at this indoctrination game. How did you ever learn how to program people? I'm curious."

"I learned from the best of the best. The master programmer who instructed me was Dr. Herman Von Heinrick. He's dead, you know. The Oracle wanted him to come here and do his mind twisting on the kids, but I came instead. I was considered his prize student."

"I didn't know. So who was this Dr. Von Heinrick?"

"I met him in Paraguay. He was part of the Samson group. You know, that bunch that was arrested in Mexico back in the early nineties. They shot him along with the other leaders. I guess it was a sort of stand-off in the hills of Sonora. He was crazy, you know. The press didn't have a lot to say about the group. I think he went off the deep end toward the last. When I was training under him in the jungles of Paraguay, he was talking about deep-brain electrodes to program members of the compound, which was set up in the jungles of that godforsaken country. He maintained that with his twisted brand of brain surgery, he could perform deep-brain implants that would allow cult members to function at a somewhat normal level, but be controlled in key emotional responses and programmed to function as the leaders desired. He taught me the science of mind control through drugs and physical trauma. Later, after I left, he developed a higher level of human control through surgery. He was a remarkably brilliant man but scary as hell. He worked with me and demonstrated how to keep an inductee drugged. He harassed them by not ever allowing them more than four hours of sleep at night, the grueling punishment of withholding any kindness, then smothering the victim with phony love and affection. He taught me the whole course."

"You must have learned your job well. You nearly have that girl over there." He gestured with his free hand toward the other prefabricated building across from the communications center where Brenda was experiencing troubled sleep. She would be up in one hour, forced to repeatedly recite her pledge to the Oracle and Gateway.

Jeremiah again gripped Martha's knee and said, "To me this Dr. Von— whatever the hell his name is—sounds like the kind of guy Dr. Frankenstein would have relished. How is it done? Not that I care to do it."

"Yeah, I guess you could say that. But I learned a lot from the man." She turned from eyeing the console to look Jeremiah squarely in the face. There was a sparkle in her eyes, a pensive look, an insight. "The brain is tricky to define. It's not a great deal different from this computer, only much more advanced. When I start with an inductee, I have to crash the hard drive in their brain. I try to wipe the brain as clean as possible, then start over again and reprogram it the way I want it to respond. You'll be surprised. Before we get through with all those kids out there in the compound, they will have speedier mental responses, greater learning retention, and great memories of what we determine to plant there. This can all be achieved through physical, psychological, and chemical responses. All of our actions start in the brain. We know that the brain is electrically excited and it transmits electrical signals. It all happens up here." She patted the top of her head and boasted of her abilities. "I may surprise you with what I know about the brain, such as the stuff that allows those neurons in your skull to build neurotransmitters, which allow your brain to form new connections. I'm involved in brain training. It's that simple. After I crash the brain . . . "

"How?"

"Drugs, sleep deprivation, love, hate, and a hundred other small but effective ways. It works. At least most of the time. Then, after it crashes, I come in and boost the neurotransmitter activity. That is where programming comes in. It is also where drugs play a part. I break through by swamping my trainees and getting the kids to consume chemical substances. Besides, I give these kids a chemical kick."

"You're a regular sweetheart."

She ignored the barb. "Today's chemistry is a remarkable thing. I let the mind duke it out with free will. Free will is an enemy to me. Free will is like unstable molecules that are called free radicals in the brain. The minds of these young people keep cranking out the free radicals, and I chemically go about neutralizing them. Certain drugs have been celebrated over centuries of study and practice to aid in mind control. The Asian mind has figured out that substances from the ginkgo tree increase blood flow and oxygen in the brain. If I control the increases, I can program better. Then, of course, there are such things as nootropics or smart drugs. Many of these are synthetic—man made—not all, but they work. They affect the nervous system. When they kick in, I get a jump-start and move these kids into a state of total obedience."

"Are these legal drugs?" For Jeremiah, such a question sounded naive. She laughed, throwing her head back.

"You, of all people, want to know if they are legal? Give me a break. Of course not. But you can order them by mail from Hong Kong or a dozen other places. With drugs I step up the communication between the left and right hemispheres of the brain. I get left-right cross talk out of these kids. Some of the drugs I use are related to LSD. We are fast entering the age of smart—I mean really smart—drugs. In the next twenty or thirty years I'll be able to do all that I want to do for these kids with drugs. I won't have to subject them to the kind of physical torment that I'm doing now. The day is coming when we'll take another human being and program that kid to go from a low C-grade brain to a bright mind. And these kids may not need to pop synthetic stimulants; they may choose to go natural. It's an exciting world we're living in."

"Maybe. This really gets you off, doesn't it?

"Yeah. Why wouldn't it?"

"Because not everybody is into your brand of brain twisting. Isn't that right? I know for a fact that some of these kids failed to come around. Right? Yes, indeed. But the day is coming, you say?"

"Rachel would have challenged even Dr. Von Heinrick." Martha's person suddenly grew silent, shifting her eyes to stare vacantly at one of the monitors. She then threw back her long, dark, wavy hair and pressed both hands to her temples as if she were weary or discouraged. She spoke without looking at Jeremiah, "Like the song says, 'I wish I didn't know now what I didn't know then.'"

"Boy, you're letting things get to you today." He squeezed her kneecap and the grip brought her full attention back to the man she knew was a paid killer. She didn't want him touching her any longer, not that sort of touch. She purposely shifted her legs away from him and slid them under the long table that held the computer, printer, and fax machine.

"Lighten up, Mother Martha. Your life's not in the pits, at least not yet."

"How would you know?"

"I found out a little something that might interest you."

"What?"

"Reuben tells me that some oriental surgeon is coming to Gateway in the near future to try a couple of experiments."

"Who?"

"I've told you all I know. Keep your ears open."

* * *

Stephen wheeled Dr. Polk into the newly remodeled office at the Sundberg Olpin Mortuary. For the past twenty-four hours, he and Stephen had been trying to contact Roy's parents in Boston to break the sad news of their son's death. All they got was a recording telling them that the Carvers were away in Maine on a much-needed vacation to view the fall colors.

Arrangements had to be made. The county would be releasing the body to the family—or in this case to Dr. Polk—tomorrow morning for shipment to Boston. That had already been determined by Dr. Polk, regardless of directions from Roy's family. Roy did have a brother in Boston who was a surgeon, but he and his wife had gone to Maine with the parents. They would return in the morning, from what little information Stephen could glean from a babysitter at the brother's home.

The Sundbergs were professional about the entire arrangements. The mortician family had been around Utah Valley for four generations. Elwood had been in the mortuary business all his life, and now his son was taking over, though Elwood was personally assisting Polk with Roy's funeral arrangements. Polk and his children had used the mortuary after the death of his wife four years ago and had appreciated the careful, loving service they had been given.

Now Dr. Polk and Stephen waited inside the director's office while Sundberg, in an outer office, took a call from Delta's Air Freight concerning the shipment of Roy's body east.

"I want you to know something, Stephen." Polk's lips were tight, the muscles along his jaw strained. He was forcing back the tears as he spoke. "I loved him as one of my own. He was so good to me. I really can never get over this. Not only did I depend on him these past couple of years, I loved him dearly."

Polk dropped his head and studied his hands, hands that had never lost puffiness since the stroke. Poor circulation, the doctor said.

"Why? Why did this happen to Roy?"

"Well, the fire inspector hasn't issued an official report, but he indicated that he thought it must have been caused by faulty wiring in the sound control room where Roy was at the time."

"But why didn't he get out of there?"

"They're still investigating. We may never know. Maybe he had the door closed and it jammed. Maybe something fell and obstructed his escape path. They seem to think he died of lack of oxygen when the flames spread. They just don't know."

"Does it matter? He's gone. If I didn't have hope in my heart concerning the resurrection, this would be an unbearable moment for me." Polk looked up at the ceiling light, bright yellow as it cast rays out from the center of a frosted glass fixture, and declared, "I'm going to personally do Roy's work for him at the Provo Temple when, at some future time, I can convince his parents that it is right. If something should happen to me, promise me, Stephen, that you will do it yourself."

Stephen had grasped the concept of vicarious work in the temple within the past year, but it still amazed him that in the gospel of Jesus Christ there was such recourse for man in the eternities—a marvelous doctrine to contemplate, especially at this moment.

* * *

"I just don't know how I will get along without him, Stephen. I don't know," Polk said mournfully from his wheelchair in the center of his living room in the home where he had lived for the past twenty years.

Stephen sat across from Dr. Polk, shaking his head and lamenting with the good professor the recent death of Roy Carver. Since the tragedy of the fire at the Center, there had been little progress on any projects. Stymied by the sudden loss of life and property, both men sat dismayed. Their world had been turned upside down.

Dr. Polk sighed with a weariness he had not felt in months. It had not seemed enough to extend his sympathies to Roy's parents and tell them that their son was the finest person who ever worked for him, and a dear friend besides. He had wanted to fly back and speak to them personally. But after the initial call, while the parents were in shock from the news of Roy's fiery death, it somehow didn't seem appropriate for a total stranger to intrude on their mourning. So Polk had communicated with them again by telephone. The body had arrived, and the family had concluded their memorial services. Polk and his staff had sent flowers and cards. But Dr. Polk remained disconsolate.

"They are reserved people," Polk said. Stephen knew he spoke of the Carvers. "And I detect a certain resentment for me and even toward the Church. To be honest, I think they have reason to blame me. I do feel somewhat responsible for his death. I was the one who discouraged him from going on to Southern California to complete his doctorate. I sense that his parents feel that if I had not interfered, had not influenced their son, he would not have become involved in the Center; and, therefore, he would be at UCLA, alive and enjoying life."

"Don't do this to yourself," Stephen begged Polk. "You have to understand that tragic events happen in life regardless of what path a person takes. You can't go on beating up on yourself for something that was clearly an accident. It was, you know. The investigating team has declared it officially an accident."

Stephen wanted to change the direction of the conversation. He had been listening to Dr. Polk lament the death of Roy for the past half hour. "It's time to get on with our lives and the projects, Dr. Polk. I need your direction on where to go from here. Do we reconstruct the Center? There is at least eighty percent of the value of the place in insurance. What do you want to do?"

Dr. Polk stirred and sat up a little straighter in his chair. Stephen was right. It would be a poor memorial to Roy to leave the charred shell of the Center as it was. He had to get hold of himself. The business at hand brought Polk back to his responsibilities. He put away the thought of Roy for the next few minutes and answered Stephen. "Okay. You're right. We have to think about our next move. I have been giving this matter some thought. The Center, as it stood before the fire, was becoming too small for the number of people who wanted to tour the facility. You and I both agreed that it was. Now, because it is destroyed, I say we sell the property where it stood, find a more suitable location with more land, and build a new center, a larger one. And I'd like to dedicate it to Roy."

"Where are you thinking of building it and with what funds?" Stephen queried, relieved to see that Dr. Polk was going to get through the terrible loss of Roy after all.

"Have you been out to the sparkling new place they call Thanksgiving Point? It's just this side of the Point of the Mountain, north of Lehi off the freeway. Do you know the place I'm talking about?"

"Yeah, sure. I know where it is. I haven't been there yet, but I know it's the place with the forest-green water tower, where they have extensive botanical gardens and restaurants. Sure, I know it."

"I did something without consulting with you first, Stephen. I approached the principal owner on a piece of property near Thanksgiving Point. Just to the north of it, as a matter of fact. I made him an offer on four acres that is part of a larger piece that he controls. His name is Raymond Clark and I understand he has overextended himself."

"How do you know these things?"

"I have friends here in the valley. We keep each other informed of things that are happening."

"You're the director. It's your prerogative. I think it would be an excellent place to create our new center."

"Think of it, Stephen: We would interest the tourists who are already swarming to the Point in touring the Book of Mormon Center as well."

"You're probably right. I'll bet locating our center nearby wouldn't do any harm to business at Thanksgiving Point, either." Stephen rubbed the back of his head in thought.

"But there is one large hoop we'll have to jump through to make it a reality," he continued. "The board will not only have to approve the new center, they will also have to give us the funds needed beyond the insurance benefits and money from the sale of the current property. I don't think they are in a mood to do that. I personally know everyone on the board, as do you. They are not in a reconstruction mode. I have already spoken to two of the members, and they think that perhaps we ought not to reconstruct a new center anywhere. They think all remaining funds ought to go into scholarships and textbook research. That board in Phoenix is made up of a conservative lot when it comes to change. We'll need all the luck we can muster at this point to get them to see things as we do."

"Well, it won't be luck," Polk replied. "It will take some selling, and I think between the two of us we can pull it off."

Stephen didn't agree. He had endured uncomfortable confrontations with the board in the past and knew they were stubborn people. They hated to see the trust pour out funds for most anything. However, Polk was also a member of the board, and he knew his way around the members politically. Perhaps he could pull it off.

The conversation switched from Roy to the new center, then reverted back to Roy as Dr. Polk somberly spoke, "Stephen, I told Roy's mother that we would pack his things at the condo and ship them home to her. Would you mind taking care of it for me? I have a key to Roy's place in the kitchen drawer with my other keys. It's the brass one attached to a key chain that says Toyota on the leather piece. Take it and hire a couple of students to pack his stuff; then you can send it to his parents. But hold up on the electronic equipment. Some of that belongs to the Center."

"His computer?"

"Maybe. We need to do an inventory. Anyway, his parents' address is also in the kitchen on top of the small desk. Would you see to it?"

"Sure. He does have a lot of computer equipment at his place. I don't know how it would ship anyway. His laptop was in his van when they dragged it away from the building the night it was going up in flames. I have that and his garment bag, which was also left in the van. The van is about totaled. The front end caught fire and the two front tires melted down, but everything inside seemed to survive okay. I haven't tested the computer he took to Wyoming to see if it was damaged, though. I'll do that this afternoon."

"When you do, take whatever files are on it and put them on a disk. He was writing up his report on the visit he made to Wyoming. I know because one of the last things he said to me before he left on that little trip was to assure me that he would make detailed computer notes on Gateway."

The phone rang. Polk reached over to the side table next to his wheelchair and picked it up. He spoke for a few minutes, then placed the receiver back on the cradle. He turned for a moment to look out his bay window at Mount Timpanogos. Snow capped, the late-afternoon sun gave it a brilliant glow. At length he turned to Stephen and told him that the call was from the fire marshal, that he was coming over to talk to Polk in person.


"What did he say, Dr. Polk?" Stephen asked, as he and Samuel walked into the living room after hearing the front door close behind Polk's visitor. Samuel had dropped by just after the fire marshal arrived; but since the marshal, a man bristling with self-importance, had asked to speak to Polk alone, the two men had slipped into the kitchen to wait.

"He told me they have searched a little more thoroughly into the cause of the fire. They are not completely certain, but they're holding out the possibility that the fire was intentionally set."

"Arson?" Meyers questioned in disbelief.

"That's right. But at this point they don't have enough evidence to prove foul play."

Stephen shook his head. "The possibility of someone deliberately setting fire to the Center never crossed my mind. I mean . . . why *would* they?"

"Still, even though it is considered an electrical short that caused the fire to start in the control room, an investigative team is probing for any other cause. That's it. But they won't say for certain just what happened to start the fire."

# Chapter 11

Samuel slipped his Buick smoothly into the center lane on I-15 headed north toward the Point of the Mountain. With Sidney beside him, he noticed traffic was light this early afternoon as he sped to make their appointment. He glanced at his watch and reassured himself that he and Sidney would arrive on time at the Dunfee appointment; actually, they had a little time to spare. Knowing this he eased up on the accelerator and glanced over at Sidney who sat silently in the passenger seat studying some notes on a yellow writing pad. From years of associating with the man, Samuel knew Sidney devoured the written word. Sid may have appeared to be like a freshman with all of his questions, but Samuel knew better. The experienced professor used his talent of seeming uninformed to acquire information. His mind was a sponge. He wasn't certain what Sid was working on; it didn't matter at the moment. He interrupted his concentration. "Sid, you asked me to refresh your thinking on when the Times of the Gentiles will be fulfilled. Surely, you must have some general idea in your mind."

"Not really, if you think I have some kind of timetable. You're the expert. I bow to your knowledge on such things. Oh, I do know that from what I've been reading the end will come when wickedness abounds. The Lord has been very clear on this point. But then, you know me. I think that in some areas of the country, strictly speaking for our own North America, we have things going on that must have been prevalent during Noah's time. I mean you talk about evil flooding into every area of our lives. Look at some of the world leaders. I suppose the one thing we haven't indulged in is human sacrifice, that is if you discount abortions that are everywhere, and legal for the most part."

"I agree, but are we talking decades, or even fifty years from now? What do you think?"

"I would be very surprised if things hold together for more than a couple of decades. I think that would be stretching it."

Samuel studied the traffic in his rearview mirror and pulled to the right as he approached the offramp to American Fork.

"I agree. I think—and these are my own thoughts on the subject—I think we will have ferreted out the righteous among the Gentiles who are going to accept the gospel, and perhaps it will be very soon. Do you know how we will know when the social order as we now know it will come crashing down around us?"

"I think we discussed it the other day. Isn't the signal that will tip us off that the end of things as we know them will be when the missionaries are called home?"

"Right. When the word goes out that young and old are asked to return to their stakes, look out. When this happens, alarms ought to go off in our heads. Red flags should go up. I really think the living prophet will alert us to the end of the Gentiles' dominance of the gathering."

"From my recent studies, the Savior was very clear on this matter when he spoke before the Nephites on his monumental visit shortly after his resurrection and declared that when the Gentile nations are corrupt beyond anything we've seen, then he will drop the curtain. The thing that will signal the end of the Gentiles, after having center stage during the gathering, will be personal and collective sinning. Am I right?"

"Who are you talking about specifically? Members of the Church?"

"Some. I don't think the members will escape the judgment when the Gentiles are brought to account for their evil ways. We know members are not all worthy to have the great blessings in store for those who are righteous. When the curtain comes down, it will be in a time of internal strife and wars in most countries." Samuel lifted his bottle of water and sipped. He studied Bender for a moment, then spoke, "There's a phase two of the gathering. As we discussed earlier, phase one is the Times of the Gentiles. You and I both know from years of study that the gathering will go on, but it will be shifted away from the Gentiles and moved to the second group worthy of the gospel."

"The House of Israel?"

"Yes, but first comes the remnant of Jacob, a people who came from Jerusalem and who considered themselves to be Jewish nationals—Nephites."

"Wait," protested Sidney as he held up his hand for clarification, "you lost me. I know we've talked about the surviving Nephites that flourished in the

South Pacific and Asia, but what do they have to do with the gathering immediately after the Gentiles?"

"In the Book of Mormon the Lord promised the Nephites that they would receive their inheritance, which is this land of the Americas."

"Why aren't they the Lamanites?"

"How could it be the Lamanites? Christ was speaking to the Nephites and converted Lamanites who had become Nephites about 30 years before he made his visit here shortly after his resurrection. There is nothing in the record that tells us he was addressing the Lamanites, or that the Lamanites were even present. He appeared in the land of the Nephites on the heels of the massive destruction in the Americas. He was speaking to the surviving Nephites on the steps of the temple when he promised them, the Nephites, that they would inherit this land in the last days."

"You're saying the gospel will be taken to the remnant of Jacob. Interesting," Sidney mused. "And that group will come here and claim their inheritance and join with the Saints?" he concluded.

"Well, many will already be converted at the time of their coming, but perhaps most will not be. They will have to hear the gospel from the worthy Saints who will be in the land. What will happen according to the Lord is a sort of invasion. The Japanese jumped the gun in World War II. They will come as the remnant and, according to the Lord in Third Nephi, they will move through the Gentiles like young lions among sheep. Things don't look all that good for the Gentiles when the curtain falls on them. Let me explain one thing the Lord mentioned in his discourse to the Nephites." Samuel cleared his throat and licked his dry lips. "We who are North American members of the Church have the tradition that the Nephites were all destroyed. This is not the case with the islanders and many of the Asian members. They, of course, feel a remnant of Jacob survived and is well and prospering today. The American Saints have a tradition, based on what they have heard and read, that the Nephites were totally removed from the earth. Yet, the Lord has said when he spoke to the Nephites in the Book of Mormon that they will receive a sign that they may know the time when he will 'gather them in from their long dispersion and establish *again* among them his Zion.' That's in Third Nephi. Interesting, isn't it?"

"Why will they come here?"

"To occupy the desolate cities and spearhead the building of the New Jerusalem in preparation to receive Christ."

"I thought it would be the Saints who return to Jackson County, Missouri, and build the New Jerusalem." Sidney looked confused as he pondered Samuel's statement.

"The worthy Gentiles and Israelites will participate, but the direction and skill, it appears, will come from the remnant of Jacob who have embraced the gospel and are leading out. There will be one mighty among them who will direct the work."

"The living prophet?"

"Not sure of that. He could be the prophet, but personally I don't think so."

They were along the stretch of highway with the golf course on their right in American Fork when Samuel switched the conversation to their upcoming visit to Dunfee. "I think you're going to find this Dunfee an interesting fellow. I have questions for him that fit right in with what we are discussing. What he's involved in dovetails with the closing of the Times of the Gentiles. Frankly, I don't know exactly what he is doing, but it has to do with mass communication. The man's generous. He's not too bad at business. With his millions he has been a real help to the Center. Amazing how these young guys can do things that make them so wealthy. But more power to him. I really like him."

Samuel nosed his Buick into a parking space reserved for visitors, killed the engine, got out, and came around to Bender's side. The sparkling series of one-story buildings spread across the slopes of the hills that divided Utah Valley from the Salt Lake Valley. It had once been a wheat field. The two men strode up to the double doors of nearly bullet-proof glass and stepped  inside the tinted-glass front building. BBDox was the multimillion-dollar, high-tech complex that Homer Dunfee had built to house his network of computer software that he had already expanded to a five-billion-dollar, research-and-development industry.

"You've read about him, haven't you, Sid? The wonder child of the new age?" Samuel asked as the heavy doors slowly shut behind them.

"I understand he joined the Church a couple of years ago."

"You're right."

They stopped in the foyer before the desk of an ebony-skinned, white-toothed, smiling, absolutely beautiful young lady. Samuel told her they were there to visit with Mr. Dunfee. She asked if they would wait seated on the black leather chairs to the right of the fountain. The two men sat down. Samuel glanced up at the dome ceiling that allowed outside light to cascade down on the white marble flooring of the lobby. It was his first time inside.

"Impressive," whispered Samuel in awe of the structure.

"So, why are we here?" Sidney asked, still confused about their specific purpose for meeting Dunfee. "I mean, what does he know about what you are doing? You say he's a friend of yours? You know, Samuel, you keep approaching everything we do as if it's some kind of military secret."

"I've chatted with him about the need to build a new Center. Then I learned he is involved in a remarkable project that deals with personal communication. I called him last night and asked if he might have a minute to tell us some of the research he's doing. Anyway, I have some questions, and you may be interested in the whole thing because it ties in with Church preparation and communication. It may have some connection to a time in the future when the Church will need such ease of reaching members. Besides, Polk asked me if I would keep up the relationship."

"Mr. Meyers." It was the voice of the lovely creature behind the desk, who was leaning forward to get Samuel's attention. "Mr. Meyers, Mr. Dunfee will see you now."

Samuel and Sidney stood and moved toward the wide, high-ceilinged hall to their left that the receptionist had pointed to.

"Does he know I'm with you?"

"He doesn't know who you are. I said I would have an associate with me."

"Oh, I've moved up in status. I'm your assistant, am I? Interesting."

The door to the office stood open and Samuel peeked in to see Homer Dunfee motioning for them to come in. The view to the outdoors brought the jagged peaks above Alpine into the office. The executive office was done partly in charcoal granite with silver deco trim. It displayed a room full of high-tech equipment of polished steel, black plastic molded chairs and a smattering of computers. In the center of the office stood a seating area with bucket seats and small individual computers on pads. The several seats were attached to a stainless steel pole. It caught Samuel's attention and he felt for a moment as if he were on a space ship.

Dunfee clambered to his feet and moved around his silver desk extending his long hand. His whole body was long and lean. At 6'5" he had the grace of a Michael Jordan. At 39, this genius of a man with sandy, short-cropped hair had an angular face with hollow cheeks that caused him to have a serious appearance in repose. At this moment, though, a smile creased back the tight skin and proffered a pure chamber-of-commerce welcome.

"Good to see you again, Samuel."

"Good to see you, too." Samuel shook the thin hand with fingers that could wrap around a regulation basketball. Turning slightly as he released his grip, Samuel reached his left hand toward Sidney Bender and said, "I want you to meet Sid Bender. We go back a long way. He's with the religion department at the Y."

"Nice to meet you, sir," Dunfee said, moving his hand in Sid's direction.

Greetings behind them, the three men chatted a moment. Then, with the sweep of his hand, Dunfee pointed to his innovative conference table and asked his guests to be seated in a bucket chair seat with small attached pads large enough for the individual computer monitors to fit on each pad. To Samuel it appeared to be like a children's play set, yet very much functional for computer-wise adults. As Samuel sat down, he felt the black leather seat wrap around him like a cozy nest. He noticed the monitor to his side; he surmised that it was intended for his personal use. The screen saver was lit. It displayed an artist's rendering of laser beams that appeared to be flashing out of a large glass-and-gold structure.

A temple? Samuel wondered.

"It's an artist's impression of the temple at the New Jerusalem. Since you put me in touch with your design man, I had him do me a rendering and we put it on our screen saver."

"I like it. You have my permission to use it."

Dunfee smiled. "I thought you wouldn't mind. I have one on disk that you can take with you before you leave. You also, Dr. Bender."

"Thanks."

"Yes, thank you."

Samuel sat like a child on his first visit to Disneyland. "Well, well, well. Dr. Polk told me about your office and the high-tech look you've achieved. Very impressive."

"Do you like it?"

"It's different."

"Actually, it's very functional. I hate to sit in meetings with my top men and women and not be able to graphically demonstrate our objectives on a computer screen. This way everyone has their own PC right here in front of them. Why sit around a solid oak table with everyone having their little pad to take notes? Instead, I prefer that each person have a personal computer to access data immediately from their own sources. All of my people are skilled at the computer. They have to be if they want to be employed at a place like this. Even the cleaning people." Dunfee swept his long arms and large hands in a wide arc. "If I ask for an update on some project, I don't want to be troubled with overhead projectors, VCRs and chalkboards. My whole objective centers on rapid communication and the need to develop the latest equipment to sustain my passion. All of my staff are well grounded in computer savvy."

Samuel rubbed the top of the monitor as if he were wiping dust off of it. "It may be a little intimidating for someone with my limited skills at the computer. I have a PC, but my range of knowledge is primitive and certainly not sufficient to hold my own in this office."

"Don't worry. The monitor is there to demonstrate more than innovate." Dunfee clapped his hands. "Okay. You asked if you could see a demonstration of what I have been doing with some of my spare time. I'll explain and on the monitor show you what's happening here." Dunfee paused. "Samuel, I too have my pet projects. Now, you understand this has nothing to do with the Church. I'm doing this on my own. And should the Church someday have need of it, they are welcome to it."

"This is exactly what we've come to talk about. I've heard about your plans to have instant personal and worldwide communications. When you told Peter Polk and me about this project, I got excited. I can see the application to the members around the world, if they have the equipment to operate it," Samuel said, his face alive with excitement.

Dunfee said, "Once we have this system functional, it can go into the hands of every member of the Church, at least as a monitoring device to keep in touch during periods of unrest in nations."

Samuel studied Dunfee's expression. The eyes so alert, so intense. The long brow, the high cheek bones, thin lips and pointed chin seemed to add up to a highly intelligent man on the go. No time for the mundane, the usual relaxation sitting in front of a television watching a game on Saturday afternoon. His thin frame seemed proof of his energetic spirit. Samuel could visualize this man springing to action from the time he jumped out of bed in the morning until late at night when the body demanded rest. He liked him. He liked what he stood for . . . in seeming perpetual motion.

"I'll try to keep this rather elementary because unless you're steeped in computerese, you could get lost very quickly. And I don't mean to talk down to you. I realize you are both highly qualified in your own fields. This is my turf, so let me explain."

Bender had said little after the introduction. He was not at all sure of just what Samuel intended to gather from this apparent genius, Dunfee. Still, he was intrigued.

"Good, now if you brethren will tap your Enter button, we'll get started."

The screen saver flashed off and a new image appeared. It was a series of lines that pointed at a small globe of the world with a backdrop of tiny lights.

"If you will study this layout, you'll see tiny objects surrounding the globe. Do you see them?"

Both men nodded that they did see the objects displayed on the screens.

"What are they?" Bender asked as if he were in a freshman course studying the novelties of space.

"Those represent satellites in orbit. Eventually, our company satellites."

Stunned at the comment, Bender asked, "Do you mean you have your own satellite system out in space?"

"Not at all. When I say *our* satellites, I mean what we hope to have within five years. These plans are being put into force as I speak. As you know, Samuel, I have been a scripture buff since I joined the Church almost three years ago. When I first came here in the early nineties, I was so impressed with all the quality young people I had working for me—returned missionaries, bishops, stake presidents . . . you know what I mean." He said this as he punched in letters to access a program he was looking for. "Anyhow, I joined the Church six months after my arrival. It was Dr. Polk, who came to see me about funding, who put me onto the Book of Mormon and its incredible concepts. Then, Samuel, about a year ago you laid out the events leading up to the Second Coming before you went trekking all over the world. I got involved with a concept I think is a direct result of our conversation. We talked about the great turmoil that is due to happen, that is if our nation, the Gentiles, fail to accept Christ and his teachings, which it looks like they are bound to do.

"Anyway, I had thought for several years that I would like to have my own highly useful set of satellites that would allow for mass communication in the major belts of the globe, so that at any time one of those satellites would have instant communication with the earth's surface. Of course, this system is already in effect, with so much satellite transmission across the globe for television, military surveillance and phone systems. This is not new; I wasn't attempting anything really new. But I wanted to take these concepts and apply them to individuals. That is, I hope to have a communication system totally independent from government agencies and corporate controls, one that will beam information from a central location to all parts of the globe for the benefit of ordinary people. I think it has potential safety features for monitoring persons with health problems, people stranded in isolated places, and a system for parents to monitor their children at school or play or wherever. In an instant they would know where their loved ones are. Each person who cares to be part of the surveillance information service could wear a patch, a wrist band, an ankle band, and it may be possible with a breakthrough in a few years to actually implant it somewhere on the person like a microchip. The concept is not new, but the implementation is. What I am attempting to do is develop this independent, private network with a handful of Church members who can afford to come in with some of the funding. Needless to say, should the time come when members of the Church want to have a security shield from the world, they will be able to communicate with local leaders around the clock and the local leaders—priesthood leaders, bishoprics and stake leaders—in turn can be in touch with each other and Church headquarters. If what may happen does happen when the Times of the Gentiles is completed, then all I can say is it ain't gonna be pretty."

"What do you mean, especially?" Bender wanted to know.

"Well, as I say, I'm not the authority on this one. Samuel knows more about this than I do." Dunfee nodded in Samuel's direction. "We know from prophecy that governments will fail; there will be brother against brother. From what Samuel has pointed out to me, mass chaos will ensue."

"We've talked about this," Bender said.

"Right," Samuel agreed. "Great calamities and disasters that may be caused by natural events will strike. It's true that unless things improve it will happen when the Times of the Gentiles close and the judgments begin. There will be desolating sickness, I suppose in the form of pestilences, then famines in the earth, earthquakes, floods, tidal waves and storms, much as we see slowly escalating now, but in greater magnitude than we can imagine. I think nearly every form of natural destruction man has ever witnessed will be poured out—and I mean poured."

Bender caught the swing of the conversation and jumped in. "I can say this from what the leaders of the Church have said, and that is that if the Saints are not righteous, or if they happen to be in the wrong places when the full impact of this terrible era strikes, it will be a sad day."

Samuel commented, "We know why all of this has to be. The Lord has told us in the Doctrine and Covenants that his indignation will be kindled against their abominations and all their wicked works. It's these evils that man will perpetrate that will bring on the severe judgment."

"I think the three of us are in agreement that it is likely to happen," Dunfee said, as if in summary. "The Lord is not going to stand by and let the world sink deeper and deeper into Satan's camp."

Samuel moved the swivel bucket seat toward Dunfee, as if Dunfee had asked a question, when he said, "I wish I knew when all of this is to take place. I do know it will come on the heels of the end of the Times of the Gentiles, when the missionaries are called home. At that time a curtain will fall on phase one and when that happens . . . which brings us to why we are here. Brother Dunfee," Samuel went on; the moment was propitious to ask, "I don't have the time fixed in my mind. We know we are not talking about the advent of the Savior in his glory when the Millennium will be ushered in. That comes later, not at the end of phase one." Samuel shook his head. He touched the keys on the monitor as if pondering a thought, then said, "Frankly, the reason we're here is to discuss these things you are working on. What you are doing seems to fit the pattern of what needs to be done insofar as all the members staying in touch throughout the stakes of Zion. If you don't mind, we'd like a little more of your inside view of a couple of your projects, unless they are so secretive it would put you in an uncomfortable position. We're not trying to steal your secrets, it's just that I understand you are willing to put up a good deal of time, research, and money to lay the foundation for some rather sophisticated communication systems that can eventually benefit us all."

"Well, it's not really public knowledge, but a whole lot of people seem to know I'm attempting to pull together a private communication network that may have merit for personal use."

"What are we talking about when you say equipment? For what purpose?" Bender wanted answers with each area of discussion.

"At some point in setting up this private communications system, we will want to break loose from a strictly commercial venture with outside investors, to have the freedom to make it totally private and for a specific use that can benefit the righteous. I'll leave it at that. The way we are moving, I think we can shift from servicing the public to converting the system to a private endeavor so long as we maintain our contractual agreement with the venture capital group. We will work that out somehow. These are all technical points that have to be thought through and resolved, but I'm not too concerned with them. I have smart enough people around me to handle the details. What I want is to make it a working system that will operate regardless of the political, social, and atmospheric conditions. We can do this if the system is owned entirely by individuals who are willing to forego the commercial aspects when needs be and simply turn it over to the Church for whatever purposes the Church cares to implement.

"We are currently involved in setting up a private satellite communication system. This is public knowledge, but we haven't touted it to the media. It will cost over a billion dollars to implement at today's prices. Of course, there are some systems in the works that may reduce the price of personal satellites, broadcasters and receivers." Dunfee shifted in his chair. "However, if we have our own satellites crisscrossing the globe with some overlap and those satellites can receive communications, either audio or visual or both, and due to deteriorating conditions in the world, should the members remain in their stakes, the living prophet and those who will be assigned under him can have immediate access to do whatever will be required to monitor and direct members' conditions throughout the world. In this way, the prophet can direct the Church from a central location. He, through his people, can guide all of us. I don't pretend to know how the direction will benefit the members across the world, but what a boon to have instant reports on conditions. I know I will feel more secure with my family knowing that my priesthood leader is in touch with Church headquarters. I would go so far as to speculate that each member will have their own, personal two-way communications monitor with them at all times. Maybe it will link directly to the home teacher or the priesthood quorum leadership. I hope all of this is possible in ten years or less."

"What if conditions are unspeakably horrible?" Samuel said. "What do you see the prophet doing by satellite communication?"

"That I don't know," Dunfee said flatly. "But I do know we will be asked to stand in holy places, as you well know. To me this means that the members will be protected. Exactly how, I don't pretend to know. But let me give a little of my thinking on this issue. My staff and I have tossed this around and have tried to visualize how the system might be employed. Say the living prophet feels inspired to direct the Saints in Argentina. Perhaps there is mass revolt ensuing. He is concerned with the small children attending school and the risks at school, or even going outside the home as teenagers are wont to do, meeting as a congregation. Whatever. What immediate, inspired advice can they be given to ward off danger? The parents can use a micro-level instrument to flow up channel to the next in authority, perhaps the home teacher or a member of the bishopric or branch president, and relay conditions. In turn, that home teacher can contact his priesthood leader and either get an inspired answer or go higher. A step higher could be to the stake president or mission president and so on. If it is a big enough issue, such as food supplies, gathering at the ward house, or whatever is appropriate, then communication can go in both directions. All this communication will be bouncing off of satellites and routed to the appointed Church leader.

"The way I plan to design the system is for private individuals to link up globally, not unlike the Internet, with final authority resting with the General Authorities. As I said earlier, perhaps this can be accomplished with a homing device or perhaps even a small cell phone to each member and allow for rapid communication home and beyond. Maybe every member will have to have their own personal com device. Maybe the bishop or branch president will issue these devices to families and individual members based on worthiness. I can see a massive private communication system that has never been tried. The cost will have to come down before it is possible, but I feel that it will happen."

"There is no scriptural precedent for this sort of thing, is there?" Bender queried.

The statement seemed not to faze Dunfee. "Oh, but there is. The Lord required each household to make a blood sign above the door in Egypt when the destroying angel came through. What about the serpent on a pole when all the Israelites were told to look upon it and they would be saved? What about Noah? He built a ship to avoid the disaster that happened. In every case the Lord provided an escape route for those who would do the thing he requested. But they had to act on some type of preparation—a sign or a symbol—in order to be saved. I don't think the Lord has closed the door on faithful adherence to direction from the prophets. My belief is simple enough to think that some form of direct communication, whether it is this type of system or direct revelation, will be in place for those living in downtown New York or in the hills of Montana or down under. So, when the living prophet directs the Saints in what they must do to survive during the coming destruction, they had better be willing to listen. And I'm thinking that such information might just come by way of privately owned satellites."

Samuel allowed his eyes to drift up to the domed ceiling in Dunfee's office before making a comment. His lips curled in thought; then he spoke, "It's interesting you would devote so much attention to this issue of communication for the Saints."

"That isn't entirely true. We are developing it as a commercial product that we hope makes a profit."

"I understand," Samuel nodded. "But how do we know what else is happening to aid the Saints? Something may be going on right now in other places to set in motion a plan of survival—food, shelter, heat, water. You name it. I happen to think the Lord is inspiring others to do their part as well. For one, Brother Dunfee, I'm thrilled with your effort. We will need every bit of help possible when phase one of the gathering comes crashing to a close."

* * *

Stephen had gathered the family to the living room of the Thorns' home. It was late afternoon, and most of those in the room were fasting. Fasting was not easy for Todd and Max. They had been doing it since last summer, but always their stomachs growled and the slight light-headed effect bothered both of them. But they did it. Max was not family, strictly speaking, but nearly so. He wished with all his heart that he were and that he were going to the temple with Todd to be sealed. He sat next to Katherine who had never fasted; in token, she skipped one meal. Fasting had become part of the Thorns' spiritual mode of life.

Stephen and Anney had already had a prayer together in the bedroom before coming to the living room to meet with those who would be going to the sealing; Katherine and Max wouldn't be going. They understood the sacredness of the occasion and were perfectly at ease knowing that in the lobby of the temple they would wait to receive the newly sealed couple and Todd, who would be sealed to his parents.

Stephen waited until everyone was quiet and seated about the room. Peter Polk, Samuel, the bishop and his wife were all present. Stephen began, "Thank you all for coming. I feel like a young groom. I never dreamed that I would be part of such a glorious event. Really, I never knew that such things were possible in life. Can you imagine the sweeping importance of this day for Anney and me? The bishop mentioned that we would be husband and wife for eternity. That's literally forever. I can't think of anyone I would rather spend forever with than Anney." Stephen glanced at Anney and curled the side of his mouth in that knowing grin.

"Thank you, honey. I feel the same way," Anney said.

Stephen turned to the side and caught the eye of his bishop. He was fairly new in their lives, but he had taken the time to walk Stephen and Anney through the temple ordinances and sealing procedure, at least as much as he felt appropriate to explain, and was the one who issued the temple recommends, though much of the instruction about the importance of the sealing had been taught at the Thorns' old ward in Lafayette prior to their move to Provo. The bishop was about Stephen's age, a large man with a full face. His smile at the moment was in complete approval of Stephen and Anney.

Stephen had asked that Dr. Polk pronounce a blessing on him, Anney, and Todd prior to driving to the temple. It would be one more sustaining influence on this grand day.

For a moment no one thought about the sadness of what had happened at the Book of Mormon Center. It was, for the group, a singular event that would not be tarnished by sadness. This was a moment when two people would become one throughout eternity. All of this Stephen and Anney had absorbed and believed with all their hearts.

Anney allowed herself the sadness of concern that Brenda was not going to the temple with them. Surely in time she would accept the gospel and be part of this wonderful event; then they would return to the temple with her and be sealed. *Yes,* Anney thought, *in time.*

* * *

"I thought it was interesting when the sealer . . . that's right, isn't it? They do call the man who sealed us together a sealer?" Stephen commented in the dark as he and Anney lay in bed, both unable to let sleep silence them after their moving experience in the temple earlier in the afternoon.

"You're probably right. I think he is called a sealer. All I remember was his name, President Lillywhite. Didn't they say he was a member of the temple presidency?"

"Yeah." Stephen turned to see Anney's profile in the faint light filtering through the drapes. Her eyes were closed. It crossed Stephen's mind that she lay there like a princess whose beauty in the dark looked surreal, as if an artist had wanted to capture the essence of charm and graciousness and used the tones of nature to achieve that goal. "You really are beautiful, Anney. I mean beyond the physical. When I looked at you across the altar and we made those covenants, I thought, *How is it possible that this lovely lady is mine?* Really, I did."

"Some of those same thoughts were rushing through my mind. I don't think I heard half of what President Lillywhite was saying. I was too taken up by the moment." Anney moved her head to the right to meet Stephen's gaze. She lowered her voice even more than the near whisper in which she was speaking to him. "Something interesting, and for me strange, happened when Todd came to the altar to be sealed to us. The Spirit—I'm sure it was the Spirit, Stephen —let me know that our Brenda would one day be with us in the temple." Anney quickly followed that intelligence with, "Do you think I'm merely hoping that it is so?"

"No. As a mother I think you have the right to that kind of knowledge. I'm glad you got that impression. I didn't, but I believe what you received. I truly believe we'll get our sweet Brenda back and in the Church. I believe it."

\* \* \*

They stood shoulder-to-shoulder in the cavernous cave that nature had hollowed out aeons ago. The limestone walls were no longer damp. Josiah, the Grand Oracle, had seen to that when he had concrete and reinforced steel beams constructed within this cave that stood adjacent to the compound and was part of the Gateway complex. Locals had known of the cave; some had visited it. But for the last five years it had been off-limits to visitors. Only a select group of commune followers and well-paid employees were allowed inside the now fully habitable cave.

The Oracle was not often depressed. When he was, he would hide away for days without allowing anyone near. It was where he sometimes secluded himself from the great challenge of being an inspiration to those around him. The small, tropical area was useful for other purposes in reaching harmony for his people.

Josiah had set aside another section as an armory. And, of course, there was the grow room teeming with plants that grew around the clock under the warm lights that helped to create the finest, most productive poppy grow-garden in all of Wyoming. The Oracle had his own source of drugs inside the cave. All in all, the caves housed the machinery and tools that made up the lifeblood of the compound. They were his prized possessions. He often came to this spot to gaze at the powerful equipment he had amassed. As Josiah stood with Reuben, a man who professed to share his dream, he felt a sense of wonder and accomplishment.

"I tell you, Reuben, there is nothing in private hands in America to compare with it. We have achieved a first-level accomplishment with this secure armory that others merely dream of having." There was great pride in Josiah's voice as he surveyed his arsenal that stood ready before him.

The Oracle's part-time military adviser was by birth an Israeli, Musrada Murma, a man like Josiah. Trained by the best strike-and-defeat instructors in the world, the Israeli-trained adviser came once a month to instruct and report. A future military force inside the compound was essential to his plan. Exercises by the small cadre of young men and young women were conducted in isolated regions of the confined area of the compound.

Lined up against the cave wall stood two spit-and-polish Hummers with missile launchers welded to their rear racks. One of the ingenious military men—who doubled as an engineer, along with his regular duties of patrolling the perimeter of the compound—had designed a fast-moving small tank and actually produced it inside the cave. Parts had been purchased by the engineer at different times from different suppliers to preclude suspicion.

Most of the equipment within the cave was in violation of state and federal law. So what else was new for the Grand Oracle Josiah? For the past two years he had been skirting the law and stockpiling his military force, small but powerful. It was a start. At this phase his military readiness was strictly defensive. If the authorities continued to leave him alone, he would not bother anyone outside the compound walls.

The fence was, in reality, a fence-wall, fashioned after the old Czech frontier fencing. Josiah wanted proven fencing, like that once used in the communist satellite countries in Eastern Europe. He had two people on his military staff who had gained experience as young officers in the East German military service. They were currently on a tour in South America. Not even Josiah could tell whether or not these elite mercenaries were as converted to his views as they professed. They would be gone for three months. But they were impressed by the cash he sent their way. That much he knew.

Concluding their inspection of the arsenal, Josiah and Reuben took the underground passageway from the cave back to the executive offices in the main building, made of glass and steel, where they emerged in an alcove off the reception room within the executive quarters that Roy had stumbled upon. They moved through the halls. All was in order. From the young receptionist who worked at a desk inside the executive offices to the young men who handled files, or the seven cooks in the kitchen, the trim young men and women who directed aerobics and physical training in the complete workout center, even to the maintenance staff, the operation was smooth to the letter.

Reuben walked along the highly polished oak floor of the executive wing with the Oracle onto the blue-veined, white marble floor of the elegant foyer and through the double doors of the entrance, which were inlaid with intricately designed beveled glass. They stepped out of the building onto the front terrace. Josiah looked up—as he always did—through the glass and steel roof of the portico held in place by white marble pillars, a startling welcome to the few who visited the compound.

There had been a light snow the night before, but two young members had already swept clean the stone walkways of the compound. The bright Wyoming sun bore down through the glass, and light refracted in a splendor of colors across the entire front of the building.

The two walked to the center of the front lawn, which had yellowed in the past weeks and was now lightly covered with a thin layer of fresh snow. The Oracle turned around to look back at his crystal palace. He could never gaze at the magnificence of the three-story structure, which was large enough to cover a city block, without a surge of pride and satisfaction that he had supervised the construction of one of the marvels of the country. There were other structures on the grounds, but none so elaborate and striking as this main building. Josiah shielded his eyes from the midmorning sun as he pointed out to Reuben the new shield the building designer had placed on the west side of the glass roofing. It was temporary, tinted plastic sheeting, which was required to protect the art gallery on the third floor from too much direct sunlight.

The building was constructed almost entirely of triple-pane, lightly tinted glass. The roof angles of the 40,000-square-foot building rose like a huge iceberg, the vaulted roof rising to a peak. There were five wings whose bright halls led off the center foyer to areas designed for specific purposes: the executive suite, dorms, recreational, and work stations. Where they converged in the center was the main focal point. The spire of the ceiling that rose above the three stories seemed to extend to heaven. A glance upward always made a dramatic, pristine impression on those who entered. It was a five-year dream that had become a reality for Josiah, who took great pride in this singular monument to God.

"Reuben, would you fetch Martha for me? I need to speak to her in my office. I have made final arrangements for Dr. Chow En Chang to arrive here in a few weeks. I want Martha to help get things in order for his eventual stay with us."

"I'll get her immediately," Reuben replied to the Oracle in near military fashion; then he paused a moment. He made a face, a question mark, and asked, "Tell me, Josiah. Is Dr. Chang the surgeon you visited in Hong Kong last month, the one you talked about, the guy who thinks he knows everything about human cloning?" Reuben's voice held a tint of sarcasm, implying that the Oracle was now moving in sleazoid circles.

The Oracle measured Reuben with narrowed eyes, taking in the witless smile. "Yes, he is. But you put your observations in such a . . . mocking manner. Please refer to the good doctor with respect. He is very skilled in genetic engineering and has consented to do a few experiments for me. I need his assistance."

"Understanding things of this nature has never been my strong point. Sorry."

"There are vast scientific possibilities and, of course, ethical dilemmas in cloning humans. I want Martha to submit to me a report on her findings for the best young man and the best young woman in the compound for further experimentation. I didn't tell her the purpose of the selection of the candidates.

I would rather she not know, at least not at this time. All I asked of her was a recommendation based on a set of qualifications: intellect (though not genius), emotional stability, personality, and of course physical attractiveness, without it being a beauty contest. She has the best information to make these recommendations. Get her for me."

Reuben left for the cave immediately, thinking all the while that the Oracle had the ability to frame issues to his own liking. He passed it off. On the chain of authority at Gateway, he knew he was number two, and that was all right with him.

* * *

"We'll have a display in the lower east corner that will depict the New Jerusalem," Polk pointed out to Samuel and Stephen, who stood behind the wheelchair. Polk was pointing to the corner as if the building were already finished. In reality, the building was still a dream. Polk sat in his chair on the grounds where the foundation would indeed be poured just as soon as approval for purchase of the new site was granted, permits issued, and funds made available from the foundation's committee in Phoenix. Polk knew from experience that the committee might simply reject his proposal. The board was never eager to spend money from the trust's account.

Samuel turned to study the location, then swept his hand toward the northeast where a stream of midmorning commuters was rounding the Point of the Mountain and gliding down toward Lehi and beyond, as well as the traffic heading northward into the Salt Lake Valley. "This is a splendid location, Pete. It will attract visitors. Just look at the traffic flowing in each direction over there on the freeway. A great location."

The land they stood on was little more than wild grass and greasewood. Polk sensed, as did the others, that if all went as planned, the new Book of Mormon Center would be housed here one day. It had been only three days since Roy's memorial services, where Polk had paid tribute through moist eyes to the loyal service of the young man he had come to love. Following the services, Polk asked to meet with Samuel and Stephen at his home. The gist of the meeting was realignment of tasks for the three. By now Samuel felt he was a vital part of this diminished group of movers and shakers for the Book of Mormon projects. He began to wonder if he should purchase a condo or something to set up semi-permanent residence in Provo. No—Katherine already had a place. His goal was to marry her. All in due time. Does this sound like Meyers is marrying Kaherine for her condo?

Polk had outlined new assignments for the two men he had come to rely on heavily. Stephen would continue to restructure the interior of a planned new Center, and Samuel would direct the acquisition of a new site near Thanksgiving Point and oversee construction when the hoped-for approval would be given for a larger, more efficient building to house the Book of Mormon displays. Polk spoke of the new Center as if he already had the full approval of the Book of Mormon trust committee, which he did not. It did not stop him from explaining to Stephen and Samuel while they surveyed the site that there would need to be more space for seating and more refined lighting, sound, and virtual reality of displays than there had been in the old Center. The other two men were in agreement.

All of the plans had been laid out at Polk's home, and now Polk and Samuel would fly to the meeting of the committee in Phoenix. It was to be held in the office that had been Thomas Kline's, currently occupied part time by his eldest daughter, Delitra. She had stepped in to pull the failing copper holdings that her father had amassed back into the black.

It was early morning. It would be another three hours before Polk and Samuel would catch a flight out of Salt Lake City to Phoenix. There they were scheduled to meet with the board that governed the trust which had been set up to administer the Center. Would there be a Center? That would be the main agenda on the table in Phoenix when the board met at five o'clock. Samuel knew from conversations with Polk that the board would meet no longer than two hours, so he and Polk would easily catch an evening flight back to Salt Lake City. It was routine to meet with the board and endure their negative input on the management of the funds that sustained the projects and paid Stephen's salary.

Samuel and Polk had been out to the site the day before with one of the principals in the negotiations for the property. The owner would sell.

Stephen now said, "I spoke on the phone last evening with the interior designer at his studio off South Temple. He assured me that it would be possible to construct a cave-like room in that far corner which would simulate the cave where Mormon compiled the Book of Mormon records. He felt the depiction should include a wax figure of Mormon at work transcribing the record."

"Well, if we can just get the funds together, sell the lot we own in Provo, and get board approval, we'll break ground here in the spring. I see the gardens at Thanksgiving Point are doing well, and the golf course is attracting some major tournaments. I think this location is ideal for the new Center." Dr. Polk patted Stephen's hand as they neared the van. "Tell me, Stephen, am I just an old fool to think this will be a great success out here? The Ashtons and others have created a worthwhile project by placing their attraction halfway between Salt Lake and Provo. It's ideal for what they had in mind. Is it right for us, though?"

Polk continued to worry over the decision. "Will the tour buses come? Will the members want to view a structure like this?"

"Sounds like you're waiting to hear a voice echoing through this valley telling you, 'If you build it, they will come.'" Stephen smiled, then he rejoined with, "You've got to get board approval before you worry about the crowds coming."

Polk flashed the impish grin he reserved for Stephen and few others. His pink, round face had filled out again since the stroke. "Right you are. Let's go get it!"

"We're loaded for bear," Samuel said from the rear seat. "I have all the plans in that big portfolio. But it will cost a bundle. Realistically, with the board can we hope to come up with that kind of money?"

"I have no real idea at this point. I'm quite certain the committee will not fund the whole thing. If it did, the fund would be dramatically depleted. Not to worry; I'm sure the Lord and you men will help me find a way to raise it."

Stephen clicked the van into drive and slowly edged his way back to the asphalt frontage road. He shook his head in disbelief. Sometimes he wondered what on earth he was doing working day in and day out with a dreamer—a charming dreamer to be sure, but still a dreamer.

From north of Thanksgiving Point Stephen steered the van up the I-15 onramp leading north toward Salt Lake City. Dr. Polk had asked Stephen if he would mind dropping him and Samuel off at the Church Office Building in Salt Lake City, and they would take a taxi from there to the airport.

"No problem."

Polk had already mentioned to Samuel that they would be meeting with a couple of the Brethren in the Church offices. He wanted to give the Church leaders a full report on the burning of the Center and bring them up to date on plans for the proposed construction. Stephen knew they had no official connection with the Center, but Polk was careful to keep the lines of communication open between all his Book of Mormon projects and the Brethren.

# Chapter 12

The committee sat listening to Polk expound on a new Book of Mormon Center. "If we sell the lot for what the realtor thinks we can, we'll make a profit over what we paid for the building and land three years ago. Combine that with the insurance benefits, and at worst we can rebuild the same type of structure. If we place it out of town a ways and have all the funds we need, we feel that an even larger site will be very successful." Dr. Polk spoke of the details of funding the project for the new Center. Samuel had briefed both Peter and Stephen on the finer points of selling the lot and buying the land at Thanksgiving Point. Polk was grateful that Samuel had such a grasp of the financial aspects of the negotiations. His lifelong friend had stepped in after the fire and had taken charge of the matter at Dr. Polk's request. Stephen felt this was a wise move. Samuel had decades of experience buying and selling real estate and running a major corporation that did a good deal of purchasing.

The foundation committee met in a high-rise office overlooking the bright lights of downtown Phoenix. Delitra Kline, daughter of the benefactor of the Book of Mormon Foundation and newly appointed chairman of the board, had convened the early evening meeting at the request of Dr. Polk. The board had not been scheduled to meet until the following month, but the destruction of the Book of Mormon Center in Provo necessitated gathering for the sake of making a decision on whether to rebuild.

There were those on the board who favored placing the money in high-yield investments and perhaps using it for scholarships. Bennett, friend and attorney for the founder, the late Thomas Kline, interrupted the discussion to inform the group that they really had no option but to proceed with renovation or construction of a new building. The question was not whether to build, rather where and when. "You see, ladies and gentlemen, our benefactor made it very clear in his instructions accompanying his bequest that there be a Book of Mormon Center and that the trust maintain it. The only matter for discussion is location and size."

Dr. Polk reentered the discussion on cue as part of the follow-up. Bennett had explained to him prior to the meeting that the Book of Mormon Center had been part of the trust when they met at Sky Harbor. "I have studied the possibilities of location and have some plans that might interest the board." Polk's speech was slightly slurred and he apologized to the group for his condition, but he insisted on presenting his proposal himself. As director of the Book of Mormon Trust, with a reserve of eleven million dollars, Polk administered the funds for all projects related to the trust.

He adjusted his position in his wheelchair and continued with his views. "I would prefer not to reconstruct the Center on the existing site."

"Why?" Delitra asked abruptly. She knew that her influence would perhaps sway the voting on any issue. She had risen to become one of the Salt River Valley's most productive, successful businesswomen since taking over her deceased husband's real estate chain. She had even branched out to Tucson. Recently, Delitra had decided to become chairperson of the Book of Mormon Committee. Her sister Marjorie had begged to be released from the family assignment. She felt helpless to make decisions and loathed being chairperson. The committee voted unanimously for the highly efficient Delitra. She was now crowding fifty, but after having a laser skin-resurfacing procedure performed two months ago, she looked to be in her mid-thirties. Polk noticed the fresh, new look about her as she sat at the head of the large oak table in the board room of the Kline family copper company that the late Thomas Kline had created and left to his three children.

"You want to know why?" Polk smiled. "Because we have a much better location in mind. We want to build on a site that is for sale between Salt Lake City and Provo. It is near a place called Thanksgiving Point, which is becoming a major tourist attraction for the region. We want to capture some of that tourist traffic, something we won't ever achieve if we build on the old site."

Delitra gazed at Polk over the top of her gold-rimmed reading glasses. "Why did we go with the old site in the first place if it's not suitable?"

"It was the best available at the time. There was no Thanksgiving Point when your father and I were looking around for a location to create the Center. He and I both agreed that it was the best available. And, as it turned out, it was. Things have changed since then." Polk stood his ground under Delitra's probes.

"I don't know," came the quiet, smooth voice of the Southwestern Museum curator. Polk knew that the man would always take Delitra's side in any discussion. She was a major contributor to the museum. He began to rattle on about the high cost of construction and how the museum had to curb some of its programs in order to maintain reserves, because a museum always requires a healthy reserve to remain operational. "We must be practical and only allow so much of the reserve to be spent on the grounds, building, and interior design."

Since the first meeting of the board, there had been a personality clash between Polk and the curator. Polk hated to be thrust into a position where he had to guard against making harsh judgments of others, but he felt he was right on this one. The man was a pain in the neck. Polk cut him off, feigning poor hearing. "If we can get the land at a reasonable price, . . . "

"What is a reasonable price, Peter?" Robert Bennett asked from his end of the table. He was counsel for the board and a voting member. He had also set up the Book of Mormon Center Trust in the beginning. Polk and Bennett saw eye-to-eye on most board issues. His question was more to clarify the costs and move on, rather than to question whether to purchase the land.

"One million. It's four acres. But let me explain the value of buying the ground we have in mind."

Delitra nodded her go-ahead and Polk continued.

"I know a million dollars sounds high, but it really isn't. Land around the Point is skyrocketing." With some difficulty, Polk unrolled the plans in front of him on the table and said, "I would like each of you to look over the plans and study the costs. We will charge an entrance fee at the gate. If the crowds come, as I think they will, then the gate will carry most of the expenses of daily operation and even allow for new exhibits that we wish to incorporate in the future. I know that the additional two million we discussed by phone earlier is a big expense, but believe me, it is not unreasonable for what we wish to build. As we said, the insurance will pay for the land and the shell of the structure. We now need five million to properly display the concepts. The building will become a major attraction. I believe that."

Samuel sat near the wall and listened. He had no authority to participate unless asked to do so. As a matter of policy he was not supposed to be in the room during the board meeting. He was allowed in mainly due to the need Polk claimed he had in case of some medical problem that could erupt at any time. Bennett knew that Samuel worked for the Center as a dollar-a-year man. He also surmised that Samuel offered a sharp pencil to the financial planning for the Center.

"Okay, Dr. Polk," Delitra declared, pushing back her chair. "If I'm hearing you right, the property is a million; construction of the building is somewhere in the neighborhood of two million; but we have to complete the interior with the latest lighting, sound, displays, and so forth. The cost will escalate to at least four and a half million total. We already determined that with insurance and property sale we can rake up a little over two million. What you are saying is there really aren't enough replacement funds to meet the over four million dollars the new Center requires." Delitra's stare seemed to bore into Polk's forehead as she made her summation. "We, of course, have to take your proposal and do further discussion, but I can tell you as chairperson that I will recommend that we augment the replacement funds with no more than a million and a half. Perhaps, Dr. Polk, you and your group ought to think in terms of downsizing. We'll go over your proposal and get back to you. We can do what we need to do in the next couple of weeks by phone and fax. I don't see any need for a further board meeting. Do I hear a motion for adjournment?" Delitra had that gift directly from her father, to do a summation that left little to discuss, at least on Polk's end.

Dr. Polk swallowed, thought of all the rebuttal he could make, looked around the table, and decided that perhaps when new plans were presented, when the design and needed state-of-the-art equipment could be shown on paper, he could request another meeting of the board and get the remaining million or so that he would need to do the Center as he had envisioned.

\* \* \*

The day after returning from Phoenix, Samuel and Sidney met for lunch at Los Hermanos out on old Highway 91 in Lindon. It was a renovated rock house that had been built in the 1890s. Now it housed the Mexican restaurant that was a real success, partly because it had mostly Mexican chefs to prepare the authentic foods of that great Lamanite culture. Samuel loved lunching at Los Hermanos. He had acquired a taste for Mexican cuisine and relished in its hot and spicy flavors.

"I've never been here, Sam. Thanks for bringing me," Bender noted with much appreciation. It wasn't the meal he had come for; it was the session that Samuel had promised him.

While they waited for the platters of chili rellenos to arrive and munched on corn chips and salsa, Bender deluged Samuel with questions about the mighty one who was to come. "Who will it be and when is he supposed to arrive on the scene as part of the gathering?"

Samuel had to speak up for Sidney to hear him over the clatter of dishes and voices of animated patrons. "Well, you know this is an interesting part of the traditions of the Church. The idea of a mighty one has sort of fallen into a traditional thinking in the Church. Most of those who even know of the phrase have long ago put it to rest. President Joseph F. Smith had something to say about it, but generally no one gives much thought to this mighty one that has to come and do a great work."

"You mean the one called mighty and strong?"

"Exactly." Samuel took a long swig of ice water to cool his tongue. "Now, keep in mind that this is solely my opinion of things as they will unfold surrounding the mighty one. If you look at the blessing that Father Lehi gave to his little son Joseph, he specified that this mighty one would come through the posterity of Joseph. Then in Doctrine and Covenants it says that a person mighty and strong will do a great work at some point in the gathering process. I believe that this mighty one and the mighty one of Lehi's prophecy are one and the same. I further believe that he will come and lead his people, whom I believe are the remnant of Jacob, to retake the land, translate the sealed portion of the plates that Joseph Smith was forbidden to do, and spearhead the building of the New Jerusalem.

"It's in Second Nephi Chapter Three where Lehi mentions that a mighty and great one will appear on the scene and do marvelous works of restoration. The scripture begins with Lehi speaking of Joseph sold into Egypt; then the next Joseph during the restoration is obviously Joseph Smith. But when Lehi was giving his son Joseph his great and last father's blessing, he told this little son that this mighty one would be from Joseph's posterity. Yet, if you look at the footnotes in Second Nephi, someone has stated that this mighty one is Joseph Smith. Wrong! Dead wrong."

"Why do you say that?"

"Because it couldn't be Joseph Smith. The mighty one will come through Joseph's line, the son of Lehi. It's in the father's blessing. I can't see it. If they say it is Joseph Smith, then Joseph Smith would have had to come from Nephite blood. As near as I can tell, Joseph Smith's ancestral line came out of the Near East at the time of the dispersion of the Ten Tribes. The Smith line came through Europe during the Dark Ages and made their way to England, then to New England where Joseph was born of wonderful parents. It's the wrong gene pool for Joseph Smith to be a descendant of Joseph, Lehi's son. Don't you see? The mighty one who will lead out in the last days has to come from Nephite lineage. I know the Lord works in some interesting ways, but he usually does it through logic and laws of nature. How on earth could Joseph Smith be the mighty one promised to Lehi's son as a future descendant when his son Joseph was born in the wilderness sometime after the departure of the Smith's ancestors from the Near East? It's one of those flaws in the footnoting of the Book of Mormon. It happens. Someone didn't catch it and stop it from going to press, and so the footnote has remained there and no one has challenged it."

"Okay. I think you're right. What would I know?" Sidney said. He pulled back long enough for the food to be placed in front of him; then he ignored the steaming food with his nose directly above it and asked, "I'm more interested in what this mighty one will do than whether someone caught an error in the footnotes of the Book of Mormon. What is he supposed to do as a mighty one?"

"It will be a vital role that he will play. Lehi said that this mighty one would do much good in both word and deed, being an instrument in the hands of God, with exceeding faith to work mighty wonders, and do the thing which is great in the sight of God, unto the bringing to pass much restoration unto the house of Israel and unto the seed of his brethren ."

"When?"

"Probably when the remnant is again gathered on this land from their long dispersion. This mighty one, I believe, will receive the sealed plates that Joseph Smith was forbidden to translate. If so, he may translate those plates and then take his people into a whole new realm of life. I believe he'll usher them in to a Zion society."

"Why that is a thing that the Church has not yet accomplished." Sidney had not yet touched his plate. "How can they do it, if we tried and failed?"

"I'm sure they will have the translation from the sealed plates, which both Mormon and Moroni called the GREATER THINGS," Samuel replied. "We never qualified to receive them. I believe that they will. For without the power in those mighty scriptures, which the Nephites had when developng their Zion, I don't think any people can accomplish it."

"Won't that require a seer for such a translation?" Bender asks.

"Certainly," Sam responds. "If you will remember, Lehi promised Joseph such a one in his posterity, one who would be a restorer. Certainly he will be one chosen of God through His prophet. We'll discuss the makeup and contents of the greater things another time. Meantime, your food is getting cold. They'll heat it for you in their microwave oven." So saying, Samuel signalled a waiter.

As Bender ate his dinner, he asked Samuel to tell him what the greater things contained. "That's something I never encountered in my studies. Where is it recorded?"

"In Third Nephi, Chapter 26, verses 9 and 10. Also Ether, Chapter 4, verse 13."

Sidney reads the three verses and comments, "Sam, that tells me something I never knew before--the very reason why the Lord placed a condemnation on His people in D&C Section 84. It's because the greater things were withheld! Also that none of the Church members fully believe or understand the Book of Mormon. Proof of that is in the withholding of these greater things."

"Exactly as I see it, my friend." Sam concurred, "That has been the trial of our faith, and we have flunked the test."

"Does this mean what I think it does, Sam; that due to our unbelief and the consequent withholding of the greater things, is the very reason we couldn't fulfill the Lord's commands to either develop His Zion or build His New Jerusalem? How can we help our brethren and sisters to know these things?"

"I see you share the same concerns I have, Sidney, but I don't know how to answer that. All I know to do is spread the word as widely as we can, hoping some may believe."

"Count on me to help any way I can, Samuel," Sidney said.

"By the way, can you go with me this evening at five to meet with Dr. Tyler? He's the one who does so much with laser light. He has done an amazing study on the New Jerusalem. Also, he's a great supporter of the Center. You'll like this man."

\* \* \*

Stephen's and Anney's conversation about Brenda had no end. It was late afternoon when Stephen said, "Honey, take just one Tylenol P.M. I know you need something to get to sleep at night, but I don't want you to take any more than you really need."

"If I go to bed too early, I wake up in the middle of the night unable to go back to sleep." Sleep had never been a problem with Anney throughout their twenty-odd years of marriage, until now. Over and over again she would lie awake and ask herself, why? What had she done as a parent to cause Brenda to bolt college and bury herself in some strange cult group, if in fact it was a cult that she had joined. It sounded like one.

They had been able to piece together some of the facts. Brenda's roommate at Redlands was the most informed person they had talked to. According to Judy, Brenda had attended some off-campus meetings where an older man spoke to interested students (and only students). When Brenda came back to the apartment that first night, she had spoken in glowing terms about this marvelous man who wanted the group to sincerely study some sort of new world. Judy had been at class when Brenda packed her things and left the apartment. The note Brenda left on the kitchen counter simply said, *Judy, Sorry to leave you so suddenly. My share of the rent is paid to December. Hope you find a new roommate. I really like you. Best, Brenda.*

Though Brenda was the topic of conversation every evening, for the most part Anney and Stephen had determined that in spite of her disappearance they would go about their daily living and make the most of it. Stephen mentioned several times how much he wished he were not so busy with the Center and all the responsibilities that rested on him since Roy's death, but he had little choice in the matter.

Anney was glad Samuel was good to step in and help. He became Stephen's "gopher" and did whatever was asked, from revising designs of displays that were destroyed in the Center fire to meeting with the Lehi City Council for permits.

* * *

Dr. Tyler held out his hand, a smile crossing his face, his intelligent, hazel eyes piercing those of Samuel's and Sidney's. The dermatologist had the same reddish complexion as Dr. Polk and was almost the same height. The major difference was age. Samuel thought that perhaps he was in his late forties, no more, as he shook hands with the doctor.

"James Tyler," the doctor said before Samuel could introduce Sid. "You're on campus in the religion department, I understand. Is that right?"

"Yes. I'm Sidney Bender. Nice to meet you, Dr. Tyler."

"Well, time is limited, Samuel. Let's get right to it. I'm always happy to talk about one of my favorite subjects. So have a seat and I'll explain." It was the consultation room they met in that contained three brown plastic-covered chairs, a small pressed-wood table, and in the center a monitor where Dr. Tyler showed CD-ROM depictions of laser resurfacing procedures for patients to better understand the method before having surgery. The two arrived after hours, with only one nurse to usher them into the room.

"You must have heard something about what Samuel has asked me to do, Dr. Bender. Is that right? I understand you are interested in my concept of light as it relates to the city of the New Jerusalem, or to the gospel to be more accurate."

"Right. I'm interested. Actually, I hope to get enough of a grasp on the events of the Second Coming to be of some use to Sam here."

"Did you mention to him, Samuel, that we are thinking of doing a depiction in stills and a miniature layout of the New Jerusalem for the new Center?" Tyler turned to Sidney. "Since not one of us has seen the city, there is a lot left to the imagination. But we will try our hardest to come up with a feasible concept of design and function."

"Jim, we are beyond simply thinking about it. We are actually going to do it," Samuel corrected, smiling.

"Good." James Tyler moved around the consultation table. He placed a yellow legal pad in front of him, retrieved his Cross pen from the upper left pocket of his white smock, and slapped his hands together.

Samuel reminded Bender, "Dr. Tyler understands that we are investigating aspects of the events that are prophesied to occur before the Second Coming of the Savior. One of the key issues or events is the building of the New Jerusalem. There has been a lot written on the subject, but I brought Sid along to hear you explain what you think the New Jerusalem, the city itself . . . uh . . . what it will be like, according to your studies."

Tyler immediately caught his stride and launched into the discussion. "I'll tell you one thing. When the Pratt brothers talked about lots and barns and outhouses in the city proper, I have to take issue with those nineteenth-century predictions. Their views of the city-to-be were certainly not canonized scripture. I think if we are looking at the twenty-first century or later, we need to take a serious look at the technology that will be present. There is no question that the mind of man will develop something we can only view from our present understanding as futuristic. I can't believe the New Jerusalem will be a throwback to the nineteenth century. Can you, Samuel?"

"No, not really."

"It is why I have some thoughts that may be in the ballpark of what to expect." Tyler licked his lips and rubbed the top of his red head. "I'll share with you what I think may happen. First of all, let me say I believe light will play a major role in the environment of the New Jerusalem. The city itself will, no doubt, employ light in a way we can't even conceive of at this time. Much of what I do as a dermatologist has to do with the recent development of lasers, and that means light. I try to heal and help people, especially with light. Through my work with lasers, I have come to understand something about light and how I think it functions in the universe. Light energy and its source are fascinating to me. I have tried to pinpoint its uses in the future of civilization, and I find it will be a huge presence in our lives. It is becoming that already. I could be way off, but I don't think so."

"I'll be fascinated to hear your thoughts on the subject. Sam says you're quite an authority."

"I'm not certain I'm all that much of an authority on light as it relates to the City of Zion, but I haven't found anyone else who has given it the time and energy that I have. So I've come up with a few theories, based on my studies of the scriptures. Are you aware that light is a dominant theme throughout all the scriptures? If you took away that one word, 'light,' it would leave great gaps in the scriptures. There is something to its being a force in the universe that the Lord has talked about."

Dr. Tyler now had his scriptures on the table, flipping through the pages. Sidney reached down and retrieved his own set of scriptures from his brown leather bag that he had set beside himself.

"The scriptures have given me a new insight into light," Tyler said. There was a fair degree of confidence in his manner as he spoke. Sidney surmised that the doctor had lectured on this subject. He liked what he was hearing, a sort of fresh approach to the scriptures.

"What is light all about?" Tyler asked, not expecting an answer. "The two main theories of light are that it is either a wave or particles having substance. Light travels in a straight line, but it can be aimed in certain directions with lenses and mirrors. And, too, light comes in different colors that are a reflection of the wavelengths. This is a relatively new discovery in the history of man. The wavelengths of various colors of light vary. For example, a yellow light beam may have a wavelength of 585 nanometers. The wavelength of light that causes sunburn is down around 480.

"Each form of light and color of light has different properties and accomplishes different purposes for people, animals and living objects such as plants. Light is not merely light; there are specific types of light for specific purposes. There is observable light and invisible light. When you place a cup of water in a microwave oven and set the dials, an invisible light heats the water to boiling point. This is called directed light. We actually see only a small spectrum of light in this world. Most light goes undetected—at least by most of us. On the spectrum of visible light, we go all the way from blue light at the top end to red light at the bottom end.

"Radio waves are light waves. They can pass through buildings and with proper instruments be picked up around the world. All of this occurs at the speed of light, which, according to our best measurements, is about 186,000 miles per second. I pose an interesting question: Is there light that is faster than what we now know of—in other words, instantaneous? I think so, though the world of science has no proof of such light. I rely on the scriptures for this knowledge. I think prayer is a use of instantaneous light from our mind to the heavens and the ear of the Father."

Bender glanced at Samuel and shifted in his chair, totally captivated by what he was hearing.

"Light as communication is a recent innovation, particularly in our lifetime as fiber optics have come into play in the communications field. Telephone lines are a good example. Computer data and other methods of communication have become possible with a greater understanding of light and its role.

"Man has learned how to manipulate light with mirrors and lenses and other polished objects. He has shaped it into focus, such as in the laser, and uses it to man's benefit. There is no way I can tell you in the time we have of all the many aspects of light in our lives.

"So where does light come from? What are its sources? I'm certain it comes from the Father through Jesus Christ. Listen to what the Lord had to say about his light. Look in section 88 of the Doctrine and Covenants. He tells us in verses 6 and 7 that Christ is 'the light of truth; which truth shineth. This is the light of Christ.' You see that truth is light, and it shines and is incorporated into Christ's being. That is why we must believe in Christ. He is our source of light. I don't care what science tells us. The light of Christ is strength and insight for each of us.

"Where can this light be found and what does it do? It's right here in the following statement: 'As also he is in the sun, and the light of the sun, and the power thereof by which it was made. As also he is in the moon, and is the light of the moon, and the power thereof by which it was made; as also the light of the stars, and the power thereof by which they were made; and the earth also, and the power thereof, even the earth upon which you stand. And the light which shineth, which giveth you light, is through him who enlighteneth your eyes, which is the same light that quickeneth your understandings; which light proceedeth forth from the presence of God to fill the immensity of space—The light which is in all things, which giveth life to all things, which is the law by which all things are governed, even the power of God who sitteth upon his throne, who is in the bosom of eternity, who is in the midst of all things.' Therefore, light is in all things."

Dr. Tyler looked up from the scriptures and met Sidney's eyes. "If you take apart this explanation of light, you begin to see that light from God is in everything. And that may be all well and good, but it is not truly understood by man, so man cannot take full advantage of the power of light until it is correctly explained to him."

"How does this fit into the scheme of light in the New Jerusalem?" Sidney probed, not wanting Tyler to get so wrapped up in the science of light that he would forget the purpose of their visit.

"It's clear to me after working with light all day, every day, that the power which will emanate from the City of the New Jerusalem, when it is created, will come through Christ. There will be great power in the New Jerusalem, and it will be driven by light. It is my conclusion that the City of the New Jerusalem will be encased in light, which will be understood by those who are in authority in the city. Samuel, it was you who said that the leaders who will be present in the New Jerusalem will have complete plans as to the operation and functions of the city and know very well how to operate every aspect of the community. I say this will work with light."

Dr. Tyler removed his reading glasses and placed his left hand on top of the scriptures, then leaned back. "I think even in the first phase of the building of that marvelous city, the Lord will set up a protective barrier. A wall will go up. We know a wall is mentioned in the scriptures. Armies of the land will try to penetrate the city, but they will not be able to get past the protective wall. The way I read it, the armies will be able to look into the city and see the activities there, but they will be prevented from entering. Do you know what I think? I think a field of light, invisible light perhaps, will be set up to guard the city. It may be a form of laser light that will be a sheet cast around the city and will constitute an invisible wall. The wall can be up to any height and even join the other side like a giant covering of light. It's possible. When the scriptures tell us that no power on earth can come up against the City of Zion and overpower it, I can now see why. It will be utterly impossible for any military might on the earth to enter the City of the New Jerusalem, unless they are given permission to enter.

"Inside the city it will function in all aspects with this powerful light source. Those worthy people who are allowed to enter the New Jerusalem will be imbued with light. As a matter of fact, it is my understanding, after dealing with light and studying the scriptures and what the Lord has told us about our bodies, that no unclean thing will enter into the New Jerusalem. I think the very power of light will repel anyone from entering who is not worthy. We kid ourselves in this life when we think we can hide our sins. Who knows, our bodies and minds may be scanned by light. Our bodies may have to become so cleansed that they can withstand the light that will be present. If not, perhaps the light will be too intense for unrighteous bodies. Just a thought."

Sidney sat with a feeling of wonder sweeping over his mind. "Then you are saying that only the clean, only the worthy will be allowed to enter into the New Jerusalem. I accept that. It's logical."

"Exactly. I think they have to be conditioned through righteousness to withstand the intensity of light that will be there. Don't confuse light with visual images. As I said, there is far more invisible light in the world than visible. One may not know why it is impossible to enter the city by simply walking in, but may be repelled and it will seem like a mystery."

Dr. Tyler's nurse rapped twice, then opened the door wide enough to poke her head around. "Excuse me, Dr. Tyler. You have a call from Dr. Dixon regarding a patient in Bountiful. Would you like me to tell him you will call him back?"

"No." He started to rise. "Excuse me, there's some urgency there. I'll talk to him now."

"I'll be leaving if you don't need me anymore," she said and stepped back to let Tyler sweep past her on his way to the phone.

Samuel and Sidney reclined in their chairs and began discussing some of the thoughts they had heard from Tyler. It crossed Bender's mind to ask Samuel if he thought they would be worthy to withstand the light in the New Jerusalem.

"I hope so," Samuel responded.

* * *

Two interviews in one day—Dr. Tyler and now the creative designer. Samuel had arranged for Sidney to be with him at both sessions. Samuel knew the designer, Hatachi, who spent long hours at his board. It was after six-thirty and he and his crew were still at it.

Bender immediately bonded with Carl Hatachi, the architect Samuel had directed to design the depiction of New Jerusalem, a key exhibit in the new Center. Samuel felt that it would only take fifteen to twenty minutes for Carl Hatachi to show him the plans he had drawn up, plans he would show Dr. Polk. They followed Hatachi to the back of his large office where three drafting boards were spread around the room. There were two young men working on two of the tables. Perhaps an evening shift. Sidney could see that the third table was covered with drawings awaiting his attention.

The three men moved around the table while Hatachi introduced Samuel and Sidney to the young men working over their assigned projects. After the hellos, Samuel immediately turned his attention to Hatachi's table with the drawings on top. He glanced first at Hatachi, then to the drawings. The buildings looked so futuristic, with swept lines and curves that caused them to appear as if they were floating in space. They joined together in a flowing pattern, like swirls of snowdrifts. The water colors were vivid, with the color white dominant.

"I had no idea how much effort is involved in creating a balance between the structures and the scenic beauty and verdant grounds," Samuel said while they studied the scenes of open spaces and the cutaway of underground networks that lit up and enhanced the plans, plus colorful patterns on the walls of the buildings. Light was everywhere.

It pleased Sidney to see the sketches. They seemed as if they had been designed by an angel. A sense of magic entered his thoughts. He actually longed to be part of that city. "What a satisfying, totally aesthetic, mind-pleasing place to live. I love it. You have captured the best possible layout of the concepts of that beautiful city of light."

"Thank you. It was a lot of work to achieve a pleasing design, but I loved every minute I put into the original Center when we designed it. Now I'm enjoying this new challenge."

"We will reserve the southwest corner of the basement to display your concept of the City of the New Jerusalem," Samuel said. "We feel certain that when tourists stand at the ropes and gaze at the New Jerusalem, they are going to see before them, in broad strokes, that heavenly city, at least what we think it will look like."

Hatachi turned on the halogen lamp directly above the table, pointed his thin index finger at the first drawing that measured 22 by 48, and said, "I have these ideas, but I'm not sure they are anywhere near correct." He rubbed the top of his head, mussing the coal-black strands. He chewed his upper lip, considering how best to phrase his comments. "Let me tell you how I think the city will look. It's laid out on these drawings, but it's a tough assignment because we have no visual representation of just what it will be like. We do have a street map layout that Joseph Smith designed, based on how he felt the city would look. As a matter of fact, Brigham Young used that design to lay out the streets of Salt Lake City. The streets were far too wide and the blocks too large when the city was first built, but today the city planners of Salt Lake City praise the wisdom of Brigham Young for his marvelous foresight in insisting on streets that are six lanes wide. I think the New Jerusalem will be a city so clean, so efficient and smooth running, that anything man can imagine as the ideal setup for traffic, pedestrian lanes, tree-lined streets and electronic facilities, in short the entire infrastructure will be incorporated into the plan. I sincerely doubt that the New Jerusalem will have anything like the traffic we now see in the cities of America. It seems logical to me that there will be no automobiles as we know them. Why would a city so ultra-efficient allow pollution or congestion with vehicles powered by fossil fuel? There will be some sort of underground system to whisk people about. I like the idea that in the center part of town people will stroll the streets like a large mall." Hatachi took a breath.

"What is to prevent the city from being under some type of force field that controls the climate? There will likely be some type of canopy—invisible, of course—that will protect the inhabitants from bad weather. If you want snow, rain, wind, or whatever, go outside the city. If supermarkets today can leave their entrances wide open and stop cold air from flowing in as they do, why can't the designers and those involved in the construction place a shield of some sort over the New Jerusalem that will maintain comfortable  living conditions? Remember, we are looking at the first phase of the New Jerusalem and not during the millennium. When they complete phase one, as you know, the millennium has yet to happen. Phase one must be completed before the Second Coming. The buildings themselves will probably be constructed of a material beyond our scope of comprehension at this time. There may not be any glass windows or wooden doors as we know them."

"What do you mean by that? Why not glass?" Sidney asked, caught up in this description of a new and different city.

"Why would you, except for decoration and design? There would be no need for glass windows if the entire city is climate controlled. And privacy could be obtained by lighting. Instead of drapes and curtains, designers can project some sort of blocking colors at doors and windows to prevent people from looking in. There will be no need for locks and doors in the usual sense. Crime as we know it in the cities will be no more. Can you catch the vision of living in such a marvelous environment? No crime, no police, no jails, no pollution, no garbage as we know it. If the remnant of Jacob return--as they rightfully ought to according to you, Brother Meyers--and spearhead the construction of  the New Jerusalem, don't you think those contractors and designers will implement the ultimate state-of-the-art type of construction? We can't even begin to comprehend how marvelous the New Jerusalem will be in design and function. The Lord will surely reveal plans of construction, and when he does, it will be a marvel to those who will be allowed to possess that gorgeous city. The whole world will look upon the City of Zion with wonder. Let your mind go and think of the most ideal setting you can possibly imagine;

then you may get close to visualizing the beautiful City of New Jerusalem. Maybe the concept of a mystical city in folklore is not so farfetched."

Hatachi glanced away from the drawings that showed surface cutaways and underground facilities, including transportation by capsule. It was fascinating to Sidney, who couldn't grasp it all at first study. "I let my mind go wild on a couple of these concepts," Hatachi chuckled.

"This will be a city of the highest technological design and function ever conceived. Of course, I am not foolish enough to imagine that I am going to depict the design of the city as it will actually be, but I may be able to design something that captures the look and feel of the city and that is what I have done for the new Book of Mormon Center."

" There is one other element. In the very heart of the city, as you see in this drawing." Hatachi pulled up the large artist's depiction of the same building that Samuel and Sid had viewed on Dunfee's screen savers. He pointed to the building in the center of the city and declared, "Here is the temple in the center-most part of Zion. Some have said that it will be a building comprised of twenty-three units interlocking one with another. It is curious that three of those units will be communication centers, according to Alvin Dyer, a past General Authority who was speaking before the student body at BYU. I have allowed for some of the current temple design to come into play. I have no idea what it will look like, but I certainly like the San Diego temple design and you can pick up some of that influence in this temple."

Samuel could easily see the resemblance to some of the contemporary temples in the world.

* * *

Thom Burton tossed the several sheets of paper onto his desk, sat back in his chair in the newsroom, laced his fingers, and made a socket that fit the back of his head as he thought about Roy. It had been a long day, with two major stories he was trying to wrap up; they were finally coming together. But the thing that pulled his mind in a different direction was the death of Roy Carver. He really hadn't known Roy all that well. They had traveled together and shared the same bus ride up and back to Wyoming. Yet, in spite of his brief encounter with the kind of gawky man, he felt some strange attachment to him, as if they had been friends all their lives. Burton looked out of the ten-story office window and noticed the lights were going off for the evening in office buildings that stretched to State Street in downtown Salt Lake.

Burton had always had a pack of friends. Growing up in Twin Falls, he understood the farming community and the excitement of a county fair, bumper crops, and small-town adulation for someone who had the journalistic skills that Burton seemed to have been born with. He hadn't always lived in the fast lane. Still, since his youth he had been an aggressive, high-spirited young man with a cause: to be the best background newsman in the industry. He was on his way.

Though he was raised in Magic Valley until his teen years, his father had dragged him and his older sister and their mother around the free world wherever U.S. military bases were located. When his father finally received the commission of full bird colonel, the Army gave him an office job at the Pentagon, where he remained until he retired. Thom was 22 by then and graduating from Utah State as a journalism major.

Never driven to marry, he took a job with a newspaper in Chicago, which was then becoming a center for talk shows and in-depth news shows. Thom was attracted to the electronic media and took a job with Wentworth, an infant news broadcasting television upstart in the 1980s. He made a sudden shift and took a job with the rising KLAS in Salt Lake City as a journalist with a strong talent for researching the interesting background stories the news show ground out weekly. It took six years, but Burton made it to head researcher and vital news gatherer for the TV station. It was a television news show that did in-depth reporting on the movers and shakers in the world of politics, entertainment, business and religion in Utah. The program charted great ratings by the early nineties and had become a stable, late-Sunday-night hit for the past three years.

Probing into personalities and situations was a match made in heaven for Burton. He loved crisscrossing the state in search of "the" story. He was an advance man. His research and investigation of personalities was always at least three weeks in advance of a show's airing on regional television. Sometimes he and his staff of two, which usually arrived three days after he had explored the possibilities and made initial contact with key people on the local scene, would move about the news-rich environment like dogs sniffing for bones.

The thing that endeared Burton to his bosses in Salt Lake City and gave him a far freer hand in the news-gathering process than most anyone in his field was his uncanny ability to get to the source of whatever news was out there. He was unswerving for these first three days of gathering information for a story and could be trusted to have the story well in hand, with all the screen drama squeezed from the locals. By the time his staff arrived on the scene, he would already have pulled together the core of the interviews and would be set to begin filming personalities and individuals associated with the news account.

He had completed most of his homework on the Mormon Center Project (as he referred to his in-depth probing of the Book of Mormon Center), complete with interviews. He had spoken three times with Dr. Polk, one interview lasting a full two hours.

Burton knew clearly that the intent of the director was to present the true import of the Book of Mormon. With that in mind, he had created the Center two and a half years earlier, using a generous endowment from the wealthy copper king of Arizona, Thomas B. Kline, a man driven to promote the Book of Mormon for the last five years of his financially successful life. It was Kline and Polk who had dreamed up ways to present the Book of Mormon to Church members and to outsiders, covering every conceivable aspect of that remarkable book. From paying scholars to study the book, to presenting carefully prepared information to groups of non-Mormons (such as the fifty college-age youth who had gathered the summer before at Park City), Polk's quest was to encourage all to discover the validity of the Book of Mormon and its translator, Joseph Smith.

Thom felt that he had under his belt a working background on Joseph Smith, the original prophet of the Latter-day Saints. He felt comfortable with his study of the current leaders of the religion. After all, he had touched elbows with a number of Mormon Church officials while gathering news stories over the years he had been in Salt Lake City. How could it be otherwise in his field, located in the shadow of Church headquarters? The Book of Mormon Center seemed to represent a concerted effort by Polk and his staff to lift the Book of Mormon from within the confines of Mormon study and allow it to expand into the minds and hearts of outsiders. It seemed not the primary intent of Polk and associates to *convert* all investigators to the Book of Mormon and its excep-tional history as much as to make students and scholars across the nation aware of the complexities of the book.

Burton recalled from his interview with Samuel Meyers, a prime mover, that the whole purpose of their drive and promotion was to offer a new view of the remarkable book and its astounding history to Americans first, then perhaps to the world. He had ended the session with one very perplexed question: Why, if they planned to reach out to the entire country with private funds, didn't the LDS Church appropriate sufficient funds to help them in their gigantic undertaking?

Samuel was ready with the answer. He explained that members of the faith do many interesting and marvelous things of their own free will and desire, not expecting to tap into the financial resources of the Church, but rather making their contribution through the wise use of their own funds, resources and time. Besides, Samuel had explained to him, the Church was committed to a century-and-a-half-old endeavor—missionary work to the entire world. They were not about to get distracted from that aim which had been placed upon them by the Lord through his appointed prophets, beginning with Joseph Smith himself. Clearly the efforts had been successful, with Church membership now beyond the ten million mark.

Burton had to agree that the Church had taken seriously the challenge to take the gospel to the world and was doing well without a great deal of public relations work on the side. He was finding it interesting to do a story on the Book of Mormon Center. Then, suddenly, there was no Center. Still, he had a story, but his boss wouldn't let him air the story about the possible murder of Roy Carver. He would need more proof before the station would run such a story.

He shut down his PC, got up from the desk, and strolled across the newsroom to the elevator. Everyone had left. He hit the lights and punched the button to signal the down elevator. He waited with thoughts of Roy still on his mind. Then, as the elevator doors slid open, he decided he would make another run to Provo to check out the progress of what he already knew was a hot story. If Roy was murdered in the fire, and he felt certain he was, then to tag it murder with arson would become a lead story on the news. He would cut some interview short and try to arrive in Provo after lunch tomorrow.

Yet, something about the whole mess bothered him. Was he simply going after a hot story or did he really care that another human's life had been taken? Was his journalist mind so focused on a story that he could put a headline above real concern for someone else? He sometimes scared himself with such thoughts. The realities of making a career, especially in the media, involved stories of horror and vengence, hate and utter disregard for the personal lives of others. If Roy had been murdered it would be the right thing to do to let the entire world know what had happened. If in the process he were to have an exclusive in the media, that was part of the job. He had been taught to look for a story and make the most of it. Yet, in spite of his ambivilence, Burton knew he had feelings for Roy. He hadn't known him all that well, but what he did know about him made a favorable impression on his mind.

# Chapter 13

Burton and Stephen had not met the first time the journalist had come to the Book of Mormon Center for a tour and interviews. At that time, Stephen had been involved with Anney in moving, finalizing his legal affairs on the house and other matters in California. Thom had called Stephen from his news desk on Main Street in Salt Lake City to make an appointment to meet at his home in Provo after lunch.

Anney was out. Stephen beckoned Thom to the Thorns' large breakfast room, still sparsely furnished.

Once again Stephen began his apologies for welcoming Thom into such clutter.

"Forget it, man. I live, too. I came to talk about Roy and what happened. This thing has me concerned. I feel uneasy. Looks like it could be foul play."

"So far there is no proof," Stephen said, a little taken aback at Thom's abruptness. He was to learn that Thom always went directly to the issue at hand.

Thom waved his hand in the air and said, "That doesn't mean a thing at this stage. I was with Roy; I listened to him on the bus. And let me tell you, something major was bouncing around in his head. He was a totally different guy on the way home from the quiet but friendly sort of fellow I took up with me. No. Something big, something strange got to him while we were at the compound. He saw or heard something."

"How do you know that?"

"Because I was seated next to him when this bully, the guy that claimed to be over security at the compound, wanted to take him off the bus before we got through the main gate. I wasn't with him all the time in the compound. I was in one little group touring, and he sort of went off by himself, talking to some of the kids there. I can tell you this, though: There was really tight security all over the place, so I don't know how Roy saw anything. I sure as hell didn't. That is, there were a bunch of strange young guys and girls—you know, in their late teens and early twenties—that I'm convinced have been brainwashed or whatever, but as far as some kind of—"

"You think Roy may have seen something to do with the youth up there that they didn't want him to see?"

"I don't know. That's why I'm here. I want to know all you know about Roy and whether or not he called anybody from his motel room, or from Salt Lake when we got off the bus. Did anyone hear from him? Where did Roy live?"

"He had rented a condo not far from here. Why?"

Thom ran his fingers through his thick, dark hair and said, "I was just wondering. Did he keep his computer equipment at his condo?"

"Some, but he had a full setup at the Center. He worked both places."

"Have you checked out his place?"

Stephen explained that he had and that he had pulled up the latest inputs on Roy's computer while he was packing some of Roy's things to ship to his parents' home in Boston. "We were asked by Roy's parents to store his things until they could determine what to do with them. I'm placing his electronic equipment and computer in my spare bedroom here until they indicate what they want me to do with the stuff. We really haven't done much over there at his condo, but we will have to move it next week or pay next month's rent."

"Have the police been there?"

"No, I don't think so. At this point they've said little. I doubt that they are handling this as a criminal case. At least they haven't told us that. I'm kind of in charge of taking care of his things. Actually, we've all been in a state of shock over this whole thing. Nobody has really looked into anything."

"It's time we did. I know you must think I'm just naturally snoopy, but I investigate a lot of things that go on with my job. If you don't mind my asking, do you have a key to Roy's condo?"

"Sure."

"Would you mind if we go over there and check out the place? Who knows? Maybe we'll find something."

"Sure, we can go immediately."

Stephen reiterated that the fire marshal refused to declare a clear picture of what had happened at the Center the night of the fire. "The autopsy shows no smoke in Roy's lungs. But according to the fire marshal, that doesn't *necessarily* mean that Roy was already dead before the fire started. Some strange things happen in a major fire and they are not sure just why he had no inhaled smoke in his lungs. According to the information we've received, no one—except those who reported the fire after it was well along—has come forth to give any indication that the fire was intentionally set. The fire marshal told Dr. Polk that they were continuing their investigation, and if he heard or knew of anything, he was to get in touch immediately. The paper says that the authorities think that perhaps it was a short circuit that sparked the fire. There was a lot of electronic equipment in the studio where Roy's body was found. The whole thing went up in flames."

"Yeah, I could see that. I drove by there before I came here. It looks like you guys have a total loss on your hands."

"The news article said that the lack of smoke in the lungs could mean that he was electrocuted and died instantly."

"The news reported that?"

"Yeah."

"Usually, that kind of thing doesn't get out during an investigation."

"They even told Dr. Polk that there are all kinds of cases where someone has died from what appeared at first to be fire or smoke inhalation, and it turns out that they died at the start of the fire from other causes, such as a ceiling caving in on them or whatever. He said it doesn't always mean foul play. Do you follow me, Thom?"

Thom did, but he had been schooled through experience to accept nothing at face value. He had seen too much of the dark side of human nature to be sure there was a simple answer. He was anxious to check out the laptop computer Roy had used on the bus to see for himself what he had written.

It took all of five minutes to drive from Stephen's home to Roy's condo. Inside Roy's upstairs office, Burton shook his head. He sat back in the office chair that Roy had tucked under his oak-veneer computer desk, the only furnishings left in the bedroom he had dubbed his command center. "That's it? He didn't come by here and work on his computer before going to the Center?"

"Apparently not. I think he came down from Salt Lake and stopped off at the Center. He may have wanted to get some work done before going home. Roy often spent late nights there. He really had nothing here like a roommate or a wife to come home to."

Stephen had no experience piecing together something as serious as a murder. It was so foreign to his whole life pattern. The possibility that Roy had been a victim of violence was too horrible to entertain.

Burton had covered crime scenes for years with the paper. He had seen some bizarre events over those months of riding in patrol cars and arriving at a shooting to see a body before the yellow tape went up and the body had been covered. It was not difficult for him to suspect the worst. Besides, he had witnessed Roy's palpable fear.

Stephen stepped over to the large window that stretched from floor to ceiling and looked out on the peaceful scene of golden trees and the brook that meandered through the grounds below him. The place was older but cozy. Roy had liked living at Shadowbrook. He had told Stephen more than once that his view of the cliffs to the east, called Squaw Peak, and the blue sky above offered a dramatic view of what the Rockies were all about. A sick feeling in the pit of Stephen's stomach caught him once again as he thought of his good friend and the horror of dying in a fire.

Stephen turned from the scene that conjured up thoughts of Roy and said to Thom, who was looking about the book-lined room with one entire wall devoted to Roy's electronic equipment of computer, fax and printer, plus assorted cabinets for book and disk storage, "I have to come back to this once more. Didn't Roy give you any indication of what had gone on in the compound? I mean . . . you say he was devastated by what happened, but surely he must have said something to give you a little insight into what happened."

"He told me he was worried. I remember feeling like he was purposely withholding something from me. He said he would explain later. I didn't just feel it. I knew he was. He was acting too strange. No. Somebody or something scared the hell out of him. I'm certain of that."

"Where did you and Roy part after the trip?"

"In Salt Lake at the Double Tree. That was the end of the bus trip. I mean, everybody got off. Roy had parked his van in the underground garage for a couple of days. The last thing we said to each other was something like, 'I'll be seeing you.' Then Roy asked me if I needed a lift to my place. He seemed nervous or something. I told him my place was around the block. I live right downtown with my brother at the Salt Arms, real close to my job, so I didn't need a lift. That was it."

"So what do you suggest? Do we drop it? We're sure not going to get Roy back. The Center is destroyed, and we haven't a clue as to what—if anything—happened at Gateway." Stephen remained standing at the window. He was too agitated to sit. He turned to look out at the green belt and thought that of all the areas in the world to die, why Provo? Provo—the all-American city with less crime than most, once listed as one of the five safest cities in America to live. Yet he did die. Was it from an accidental electrical shock . . . or was he murdered by someone?

"You know what my gut feeling is, Thom?" Stephen ventured, continuing to gaze at the beautiful scene. "I think Roy was killed." Stephen even startled himself that he could say this so frankly. "I think someone set the fire to make it look like an accident. And what's more, I think it was carried out by some lowlifes from Gateway."

"That's a pretty strong statement to make," Thom said uneasily. "You've had more time to piece this thing together than I have. I don't know. Why aren't you getting a little more action from the fire marshal?"

"They move with great caution. I'm merely telling you my unsubstantiated impression of what's happening," Stephen said. "I do think something happened that was serious enough for the compound people in Wyoming not to want Roy to divulge it."

Burton glanced over Stephen's shoulder at the window and said, "Thought you said you cleared all of Roy's messages this morning."

"I did," Stephen said, turning to look in the direction of the answering machine, which sat next to the printer.

"It's flashing. Shall I replay the message?"

"Sure, just hit that little white button on top."

The voice they heard was crackly and nervous, that of a boy leaving puberty, not yet mature enough to have masculine vocal chords. " . . . It's noon, November 24. Uh . . . you may not remember me. I'm calling from a pay phone. Pick up if you're there. I need to talk to you. I can't stay here—I escaped. I need somebody to help me. I don't dare go to the authorities. I don't trust anybody. Can you call me back as soon as you get in? The number here is 307–624–6668. I will return to this pay phone at three this afternoon, then at five, and wait for it to ring. Please call me. Please!" The last "please" came out in a high-pitched, pleading tone.

"Play it again," Stephen said breathlessly, hovering over the answering machine. Burton leaned back and let him reach over and rewind the machine, then punch the replay button.

They heard the frightened voice of the kid a second time. Burton had his notebook and pen in hand and jotted down the telephone number, recognizing the area code and prefix. The guy was calling from Jackson Hole. He grabbed the receiver and punched in the numbers; he let the phone ring eight times before he replaced the receiver.

"It's only two forty-five; he said three. We wait fifteen minutes."

"Yeah, you're right."

Not since he was a child waiting to go with his family to Ely for the day to a movie and shopping had Stephen watched the clock so closely. He had forgotten how long fifteen minutes could be. It was like waiting for water to boil.

"It's two minutes to three. Let's try it." Burton could wait no longer. In the interim they had discussed repeatedly who the voice might belong to. Who would Roy know in Jackson Hole? From what the boy said, both Stephen and Thom were in agreement that it had to be one of the kids from the compound. Roy must have met someone while he toured the place. But the boy sounded so young and Stephen knew he had to be at least 20 years old to have been in Gateway. Thom was puzzled. He couldn't see Roy getting overly friendly with anyone. And how come the kid trusted Roy if Roy had only casually met him? Where did he get Roy's number, anyway? It didn't matter. They were ready to call.

Burton put the phone on speaker and called again. They heard the pay phone buzz once and a voice came on the line, "Yeah?"

Stephen spoke, "Are you trying to reach Roy?"

"Roy? Was he in Jackson this weekend?"

"Yes. Matter of fact, he was. . . . Ah, this is Roy's good friend. Roy's not here right now. Can I help?"

Silence. Had Stephen scared him off? He tried again.

"Hello. I want to help you. I'm taking Roy's messages as a favor to him. He's not here at his place. I'm his best friend; you can talk to me."

"I want the guy who was in Jackson."

Stephen took a breath. " . . . Well, . . . Roy is dead." He finally blurted out the words. He wanted to help the kid and hoped that being candid would do it.

The phone went dead.

Stephen shook his head at Burton. He pressed the off button on the phone and slowly straightened up, putting both hands on his hips and shaking his head, thoroughly depressed. "I scared him off."

Burton studied the phone without comment.

"Man, I scared him," Stephen said again, angry at himself. "I'm sorry. I thought . . . Why on earth did I tell him Roy was dead? The kid's gone ballistic. He's running and we'll never catch up with him. He knows something about what happened. Why didn't I come in with a fatherly voice? Why . . . "

The phone rang. It seemed inordinately loud. Burton grabbed it, then handed it over to Stephen. Stephen cautiously said, "Yes?"

Again Burton punched the speaker button to listen in.

The same voice came on. "How do I know you are Roy's friend?"

"Because I'm here in his study taking care of some of his things. Can I help you? You can check me out if you want to call a couple of people in the next few minutes: my wife, my boss . . . "

"You say Roy's dead?" he asked incredulously. "They killed him." His voice became bitter.

"Who killed him?"

Silence on the line. Stephen could hear nothing. "Yes, he died in a fire that we think was set by an arsonist."

"They killed him, and they'll kill me, too."

"No, they won't!" Stephen was desperate to keep the boy on the line. "We can help. Listen. There is someone else in the room with me, and he is listening to our conversation. Don't hang up, okay? We really and truly are your friends, and we were friends of Roy's. I hope you believe me, because we just want to help."

Stephen and Burton spoke to the young man until a programmed voice informed the caller that three minutes had expired. Stephen told the boy to hang up and he would call him right back. They reconnected and made arrangements. Burton calculated in his head about how long it would take to drive from Provo to Jackson Hole, then arranged for a location to pick up the young man. It would be a busy shopping mall at the local Albertsons food store. Stephen explained that they would be a couple of guys in a new, white Jeep Cherokee.

"Oh, by the way," the voice added cautiously, "so you'll know me, I have red hair."

Stephen paused at the door leading to the stairs of Roy's condo. He grabbed Burton by the arm and said, "You know, I'm all for picking up this young man, but we have no experience at such things. He is desperate for help. Don't you think we ought to call the authorities in Jackson Hole and have them get involved in this?"

Burton was suddenly impatient. The very thought that they would involve the police at this early stage of the game was not his style. "Stephen, I understand your concern, but what happens to this kid if the police blow it? One, he will bolt as soon as the cops arrive. We have to be the guys to pick him up. He's primed to leap into a white Cherokee. After we get him into the Jeep, we could turn him over to the cops, but what will they do? They'll contact the Oracle, and he'll have a ready-made story with ten witnesses that the kid stole something, or that the kid killed someone, or that the kid is not well—whatever. Before we ever get any information out of him, the authorities will have him locked up. And, believe me, the Oracle will be notified. Think about it. If you want information about what happened here—Roy's death, the burning of the Center—you'd best go along with me. Trust me. I know what I'm doing. I have covered so many police-involved situations that went to hell that you don't want to know."

"It's still a pretty risky thing, going up there and getting involved with someone neither one of us has met."

"You have just hit upon the very spice of life. We don't know. But, by hell, we are about to find out." What Burton didn't discuss was the tremendous story that could come his way out of this whole wild chase. He could smell a good story. If he had to make it happen, so be it.

"Okay, let's get going."

"Right. Now you're cookin'." Burton's face broke into a childlike grin. It was a smile, Stephen surmised, that had opened some pretty rusty doors.

Using his cell phone, Stephen quickly made two more calls, one on the way to the Jeep and another when he climbed inside: One to Anney to let her know they were taking off for Jackson Hole and would stop at the house for a second to pick up a couple of heavy jackets, and maybe a sandwich or two. Anney assured him she would have everything ready in ten minutes. She also telegraphed her deep concern for their safety before hanging up. The second call was to Dr. Polk. He was not at home. Stephen remembered that his daughter was dropping by to take him shopping. He left a message on Polk's machine, telling him what they had learned and that he and Burton were headed for Wyoming to pick up the kid, that he would call Polk on the cell phone from the car while they were traveling.

* * *

Samuel was glad to get out of his small apartment for a few hours. It was so confining. The small living room, mini kitchen and the tiny bedrooms were taking their toll on his sense of space and comfort. He knew he could always go home to the large house that he had loved so dearly with his deceased wife, but he had chosen to help with the project, and stay he would. Besides, Katherine was here in Provo, at least for the time being. He would stick it out.

He pulled on his light jacket and was headed for the front door—the only door—when the phone rang. "Samuel, I've gone over your report," Sid Bender said. "I wonder if we could get together fairly soon. I have a plethora of questions for you."

"Sure, when is it convenient for you to talk?"

"Right now, if you have a minute."

"Well, . . . okay." Samuel had not been planning on a phone discussion, but how could he turn down someone so eager to learn? A good walk could come later.

"My interest is to get a little clearer understanding from you about your discussion of what you call the 'Zion of Enoch' in relationship to the greater things that have been withheld from us in these latter days. I'm specifically referring to Moses 6:46 where Enoch was reading to his people about the Book of Remembrance."

"What is your question?"

"I . . . have never associated that reading with the greater things. You mention that the writings of the Book of Remembrance are included in the greater things that are inscribed on the sealed plates."

"That's right. However, I said they *may* be. It just seems logical to me that they are. Doesn't it to you?"

"Oh, I'm merely a student asking the questions. You seem to have the answers. Tell me, what do you think was contained in that marvelous Book of Remembrance? Evidently, when Enoch read from the book to his people they were overcome by its power, or as the scripture says, 'And as Enoch spake forth

the words of God, the people trembled and could not stand in his presence.'
Pretty powerful words."

"Sid, if you recall, there were other writings that were extremely powerful.
You recall the lament of Moroni when he wrote: 'Behold, thou hast not made
us mighty in writing like unto the brother of Jared, for thou madest him'—the
brother of Jared—'that the things which he wrote were mighty even as thou art,
unto the overpowering of man to read them.' That is powerful."

Samuel could feel the interest that Sid was projecting through the phone.
He felt the conservative professor was too steeped in accepted doctrine to admit
it, but he was coming around. "It's the writings of John that are mentioned in
the ninety-third section of the Doctrine and Covenants. I'll quote it, though I
know you know it, 'And John saw and bore record of the fulness of my glory,
and the fulness of John's record is hereafter to be revealed.'

"'And it shall come to pass, that if you are faithful you shall receive the
fulness of the record of John.' Moroni also speaks of obtaining John's record
in Ether 4:16. We haven't been that faithful, apparently, because we sure don't
have that record yet. I think it's also part of the greater things we have to look
forward to possessing before we can become a Zion people and ready to head
for the New Jerusalem. I think we kid ourselves if we think the Lord will allow
those records to be placed in our hands before we are ready to receive them.
They are too powerful for us to withstand the impact. Look what happened to
the people in the time of Enoch. It knocked them over. They couldn't stand in
his presence because they were not spiritually prepared to do so. Do you really
think we are any different?"

Bender quietly said, "You have a point there, Samuel. Yes, in fact, you do."

* * *

Katherine had asked Samuel to drop by and help her decide which of the
two recently arrived Le Caron paintings she had purchased a month ago at the
open auction at a new  art gallery in San Francisco should hang in her
townhouse in Provo. Samuel had protested that he knew  nothing about art and
that he didn't want to be blamed for selecting a piece she might end up
disliking. Katherine, being Katherine, insisted that he come by and help her.

Much to Samuel's delight, one of the paintings was set in the Orient. The artist had spent several years in Guam and had captured the simple beauty of nature in the rice fields.

Samuel expressed his pleasure and chose the first of the two that Katherine had displayed in the living room. She had covered each with a large bath towel and uncovered the second only after Samuel had commented on the first and how he loved the gentle hills in the background of a rice paddy at sunset. He had seen a field exactly like that in Japan.

"There you go. I knew you had taste and appreciation. It's your painting, Sam. I bought it with you in mind."

"What?"

"Yes. I want you to have it. I bought one for me and one for you."

Samuel was always surprised at this lady's interesting methods of expressing her friendship. Always her own person, she gave her own unique little twist to everything she involved herself in.

"Now sit down. Can we talk a minute?"

"Sure." Samuel moved to the sofa directly in front of the flickering fireplace. The room was comfortable and tasteful, the upholstery and rugs coordinated in vivid cranberry, hunter green, and navy blue. It set a warm but vital mood.

Katherine pulled an ottoman close to where Samuel was seated on the sofa and sat down gracefully. With the coy look of a teenager in love, she asked, "What do you really think of me usurping your territory?" She was not usually one to care that someone might find her a little pushy (or as she had learned in London, cheeky). She had pretty well done as she pleased in the past, and it was doubtful that she would change at such a late date in her life. No, she would do whatever was honest and right for her, though she was sensitive to people's feelings if they could be hurt by her actions. She felt few had been in the past.

Sam looked puzzled, shocked. "Why would you ask such a question? Remember, it was I who asked you to come up and be with us and get involved in some of our projects."

"Yes, you did ask me. But if I recall, you meant for me to come visit for a couple of days, not become a part-time resident, which I have done and deliberately so. I like it here near my family. I also love the mountains at certain times of the year. And, for your information, I sort of enjoy being around you." Katherine made her declaration with an impish grin on her face and determination in her voice, all in keeping with her direct way of facing life and informing friends of exactly what she intended to do and why.

"I liked that last part."

"What part?" Katherine feigned innocence.

"That you enjoy being with me. I can't tell you how much I enjoy being with you." Sam pulled Katherine around to face him and rubbed his hands lightly up and down her slender arms as they sat looking at each other.

Suddenly, he broke into a chuckle and nodded his head.

"What's so amusing?" Katherine persisted. "Did I say something I shouldn't have?"

"Oh, my dear . . . " Meyers said with a husky voice, placing Katherine's palm against his face with total satisfaction. He had to get up. How many times had he counseled young men on when to leave before things got too involved? He settled back for a moment. "I was just thinking how strange it is that the two of us, both beyond the usual dating age . . . yet I feel so much warmth and affection here. It's remarkable. I never thought I would ever let my heart go to another."

"Nor I," Katherine said softly, staring into the fire with a faraway look. She turned back to hold Samuel's eyes with her own. "My former husband fulfilled many of my needs. But lately I am beginning to feel that it is possible for more than one person to fulfill the longings of the heart. Do you understand what I'm trying to say? I don't love him any less, but somehow . . . my heart is not as limited as I thought. You have done that for me. You really have. Wherever our relationship flows, I want you to know, Sam, that you have removed some of the sadness from life and made me a much happier person. Thank you."

Samuel stood up. For sure it was time to leave. He longed to stay, but good sense persuaded him to begin moving toward the front door. This woman was entirely too vulnerable, too feminine—too desirable. He knew the power of his hunger if he surrendered to its will.

Besides, he had promised Stephen that he would meet with him to go over blueprints on the building Polk was so eager to build. It would need certain types of wood, and Samuel knew wood, at least lumber for construction.

"I really hate to go, but I do have a job to do—not that I expect to get paid, but I told Stephen I would come right back to his place and help select . . . What?"

Katherine was smiling and running her index finger along Samuel's cheek. She moved close to him when he stood. "Anney warned me about you," she murmured.

"What do you mean?"

"I mean that your Puritan upbringing would not allow you to remain alone too long with a woman. She said that Mormon missionaries cannot be alone with a person of the opposite sex. It goes against their moral code."

"Well, that may be true for a missionary, but I'm not a missionary. Do I look like a missionary?" he laughed, rubbing his gray hair with embarrassment.

"Yes." Katherine reached up and teased his hair, pulling several strands down his forehead. "Yes, yes, yes! You do, Samuel Meyers. You are as wholesome and clear eyed as every young missionary I've ever seen, and I love you for it."

"Well, that's settled," Samuel laughed, high color flooding his face. "I'm off-limits to beautiful women when I have no companion. This missionary has things to do."

Leaning close enough to breathe Katherine's fragrance, he kissed her gently and said, "I've done my duty, Ms. Moore. I came as I was commanded; I've been charmed and bribed, and I love it."

* * *

Max came dragging into the apartment with Todd. He had talked to Anney about Brenda. He felt responsible for so much concern over her disappearance. Their apartment was on the south side of UVSC. There were sweaters and towels on the unmade beds, books scattered on the floor surrounding the computer center. In the kitchen, where Todd always migrated first, dishes were on the counter and in the sink. Max and Todd had promised each other before they left for class that morning that they would clean up the place before cutting out for the evening. They both knew it was time to make good on their promise.

Max watched Todd open the small refrigerator door and stare at the leftovers. Most of the food moldering inside was from Todd's mother. She often sent him home with plates of steamed vegetables, pot roast and gravy, and whatever else was left over from their table. Todd was in no mood to warm it up. "Hey, Max. I wish we'd taken Mom up on her offer to feed us dinner. I'm so stupid."

"Forget it. Your dad isn't going to be home, so why put her to the extra work? Think, Todd. You expect a lot of your mother. Why do you do that?"

"Hey, cool it. She is my mother and she did ask us to stay for dinner. What's bugging you, anyway?"

Max frowned. "Nothing."

"Something is. What? If I've said something to tick you off, I'd like to know."

"It's not you. It's me." Max rubbed his eyes with both hands, then shook his head. "Your mom is so upset about Brenda. She can hardly think of anything else. I have some of those same feelings. In fact, I feel it's my fault she just up and quit school. I led her along all last summer, then dropped her. I thought we had a thing going; then I got this overwhelming impression that I must serve a mission. I want to serve a mission. But Brenda was not for that. I feel like she has joined some far-out group just to get even. She was very upset with me."

Todd closed the refrigerator door and walked into the living room/ bedroom and scrunched down on the black bean bag he had brought from home when they rented the apartment. "Oh, Max, Max. Don't do this to yourself. It isn't fair to you, to me, to my parents, or even Brenda for that matter. How do you know what was going on inside her head when she joined some crazy bunch or whatever she did? Snap out of it, man. You're totally wrong. Wrong, man. Wrong."

Thoughts of Brenda and her strange actions weighed heavily on Max. Just picturing her sweet face when she had told him she loved him caused his heart to ache. It was his fault. He knew it was. She had felt rejected when he wanted to postpone their plans to marry until he could serve a mission. He should have been more sensitive. How could she have understood his feelings for the Savior, his surety that the Lord wanted him to serve a mission? She didn't know what she believed. But deep inside, Max knew there were lots of other people out there who were feeling as lost and unloved as he had felt, and he yearned to tell them they could find real joy in the gospel of Jesus Christ. If he had married Brenda, she would never have gone away seeking something else or tried to hurt him. What a mess he had made of everything.

# Chapter 14

Brenda returned from the bathroom as Martha moved swiftly along the hall. Their eyes met. Brenda felt alive and invigorated at the moment. She had gone two days without a shot; then she had become distraught an hour ago, begging for a hit. She had tried to go as long as possible without giving in to Mother Martha.

Sometimes Mother Martha could be so friendly, so warm and solicitous; then, as she had done the night before, she would fly into a rage. Why? It puzzled Brenda. However, many things puzzled Brenda about her strange situation.

"Are you feeling better now, honey?" Martha chirped as if they were best friends and she were sincerely concerned about Brenda's welfare.

Brenda stopped in the center of the hall and glared at Martha as the therapist came closer with a grin on her face. Brenda blurted out, "Why are you doing this to me?"

"What, dear? What are you talking about?"

"You know what I'm talking about. One minute you're so sweet and the next you become a tyrant. What are you doing?" Brenda wanted to grab the woman and shake her violently, but she was afraid she would be punished—she might never get another shot—so she backed off. "I just want to know what's going on. Why are you leaving me for a couple of days at a time? You lock me in my room and . . . "

"You're not locked in your room now. We worry about you hurting yourself when you're in one of your moods. When you are begging for the stuff, you really have an attitude. I can't let you harm yourself. Do you understand?"

Brenda looked down at the off-white tile floor. Then she glanced up and met Martha's cheerful face. "Something is happening to me. I don't like what is happening, especially when I'm all alone and suffering."

"Suffering?"

169

"Yes. You know that I am." Brenda swung her head from side to side, exasperated. "I want to leave; I just want to leave. You can keep my clothes. Just give me shoes and a jacket. I'll call my parents and they'll come pick me up. I want out."

"Now, honey. You know you vowed to the Oracle that you wanted to remain with the group forever. Surely you don't think we can spend the time and money we have spent on you over the past few weeks and have you simply walk out the front gate. You are one of us. You are one of the winning people of this world." Martha spoke with feigned sincerity. The truth was, she was having some of the same feelings. Only she knew how to curb the thoughts of leaving.

"You feel fine now, don't you?" she continued. "You stay with us. You would regret leaving. It would hang over your head the rest of your life if you left now." Martha knew Brenda was going nowhere. She knew the rules and knew she had to obey.

"Sure, but I know you're going to leave me alone in that room again. I hate it. And besides, how come I can't go swimming anymore, and why are the doors locked? Every door in this building is locked. I didn't come here to be a prisoner. What's going on?"

Martha reached out her hand and took Brenda by the arm and said in her most soothing tone, "Honey, we are preparing you for great things. You must learn to sacrifice. You are about to learn how to give yourself totally to this marvelous movement. It is my job to teach you how to endure pain. You have to appreciate the sacrifice before you reach the joy that the others in this magnificent sanctuary have reached. You will be free one day; and when you are, you will give great service. Don't spoil it by asking too many questions. It is part of your test to see if you can become one of us."

"You're not listening. I want out! Do you hear me?"

"As I said, honey, that is no longer an option. You made the commitment to the Oracle himself, and now you have to measure up. Be patient, my dear. Be patient."

In the two years Martha had been at the compound, she had seldom met the resistance in a recruit that she saw in Brenda. Most, once they were on medication and had undergone the "test" that broke their spirits, especially when they were subjected to sleep deprivation, tended to cooperate for the reward of sleep and injections. Not so with Brenda. She should have come around by now.

It wasn't Brenda that bothered Martha, however. Her own strange feelings were threatening to engulf her. She had begun having second thoughts about programming someone so completely unwilling to join the group in the compound. There was a spirit of resistance in this young woman that forced reluctant admiration from Martha, a trait within herself that had not surfaced in years. Brenda was the first inductee in a long while to prick Martha's seared conscience and cause her to wonder at the whole scheme of things going on about her.

Surely this edgy feeling of compassion for another human being would dissolve. That's what it was. Martha knew she had to get control of her emotions—very strange emotions. Brenda's resistance seemed to be exploding at the very time when Martha needed to bolster her own resolve to continue to program the youthful members of the compound, and most especially this Brenda. She knew she had to get a hold on herself to continue to be the professional the Oracle expected of her. There were others being programmed. She had to regain control. Yes, she did have emotions, whether Jeremiah thought so or not.

* * *

When Samuel pulled into the circular driveway at Stephen's, the white Jeep was parked directly in front of his garage, and the front door to the house was wide open. Stephen suddenly came out with an ice chest in hand and shouted "Hi" to Samuel. Burton followed with two pillows and a couple of blankets. The air was cool and the afternoon sun had rendered all the warmth it intended to expend for the day.

"Hey, Samuel, you're just the person I need to talk to." Stephen explained about the strange call that had come from Jackson. Samuel listened. "We have no choice. We told the kid we would come and get him."

"Then what do you want from me?"

"We want you to go with us. I'm sure the kid is an adult."

"Burton says that all the kids are in their twenties," Samuel said. "The official report given the journalists indicated that when they were invited to the compound."

"So this young man has the right to make up his mind whether or not to get out of Jackson Hole with us. But he could probably use some wise counsel, and you're just the man to give it."

"We're going after him," Burton chimed in excitedly. "He needs help."

Samuel sat in the center of the rear seat and leaned forward, arms resting on the back of the front seats so he could hear all the details. When he had heard where Stephen and Thom were headed, he was glad to go along. He had used his cell phone to inform Katherine about his sudden change of plans. He would be home too late to call, maybe not before two in the morning. He would sleep in the Jeep part of the way.

Katherine wondered what could be so important that one minute he was to help Stephen on some blueprints and the next he was on his way to Jackson Hole. "I hope the weather is good. I'll be watching the weather report on the ten o'clock news so I can really worry if it's bad," she said.

"You do that," he laughed.

"Samuel."

"Yeah?" he replied softly into the mouthpiece.

"Would you call me when you get back?"

"It'll be very late. You'll be asleep."

"I don't care. Call me the minute you get within twenty minutes of Provo. Please?"

"You do like to punish yourself. It's not as if we are headed to the other side of the world. Okay, I'll call. Bye."

Samuel shut the speaker over the small, hand-held instrument, slid it into his blue-plaid shirt pocket, and began asking questions. He wanted information.

"What do you know about this Oracle, Thom?"

Thom Burton turned to meet Samuel's eyes. "I've been trying to get a handle on this self-styled prophet of Gateway, and I've come up with a rough profile. I got some of it from information sources I have on line, and some from a journalist friend of mine, but I'm not sure all the data I have collected is accurate. Someone like the Oracle has so many warts and scars of past activity that all a guy like me can do is try to piece together some of it. I do know this: He's smooth. Man, is he smooth. I met him when I was with Roy at the compound. He told us at a luncheon meeting—he came by to grace us with his presence—that he planned to create the ideal community for mankind, that his

Gateway was to be a model of perfection for the world to see and emulate. Whenever I hear guys talk like that—and in my business I see a few—I get concerned. You know Hitler was convinced that he had an inside track on the way all men should pattern their life. He was positive he had all the answers. Scary."

Samuel and Stephen were attentive and highly motivated. They had little, if any, evidence that the Oracle had had Roy killed . . . but both had an uneasy feeling. For his part, Stephen was gripped with terror.

Burton gave a rundown on the Oracle from memory. He had done his homework. His curiosity had been sparked by Morris Turnbull from Oakland. What he had learned didn't contain total proof of misdeeds, but close enough for him to sense that they were dealing with a fanatic, a man who felt that God had given him a special charge to the world to fit his own concepts of right and wrong. Thom told them how bright the Oracle was, how he had used his family's wealth to build Gateway. He had recruited, as nearly as Burton could deduce, an inner staff of henchmen and a membership of near-perfect, white young males and females as his followers.

"As I said, a guy like the Oracle is a loose cannon. He could go over the edge at any time. Jones did in Brazil. That's why we've got to get this red-headed kid. We not only save him, but he becomes our key to putting this Oracle away."

Samuel wondered aloud why they weren't contacting the police in Jackson Hole. As with Stephen, Burton explained that first they needed to talk to the kid, then contact the authorities. Not the other way around. He might bolt, or be eliminated like Roy had been. Samuel saw the sense of Burton's plan.

It was a four-hour drive at best to Jackson Hole. They planned to take the route north through Rexburg and across the Uintah Range and drop down into Jackson Hole by six-thirty, well in time to make the shopping center by seven and pick up the frightened kid.

"Back to this Grand Oracle Josiah," Samuel said. "Stephen, do you remember studying the Book of Ether in the Book of Mormon? At times, the civilization of the Jaredites got caught up in secret combinations and actually made pacts with Satan."

Samuel looked toward Burton who was listening to this comment but making no judgment. He always remained as neutral as possible in any religious discussion.

"The writings of Ether tell us that one Akish, a friend of King Omer, actually took an oath to follow Satan. It's in chapters eight and nine of the book of Ether. It tells us that Jared, King Omer's son, rebelled against his own father. Jared offered Akish his daughter, if he would bring him the head of King Omer, his father. King Omer escaped, so Jared became king. Akish was able to gather a sizable following because he was good at flattering and using cunning words to gain their support, and had them kill King Jared. You tell me that this Oracle is smooth. I think he is able to flatter people. Akish made his people take an oath that they would follow him no matter what happened.

"When they agreed to follow the administered oaths, which had been around from times of old, they became part of a secret group. The book tells us that those were the oaths that Cain administered, and we know that Cain was a murderer. How did he get these oaths? They were written, and it says they were kept by the power of the Devil. The oaths brought forth by the Devil had real purpose: Any man who administered them was seeking power. He would stoop to plunder, lie, and murder, and was willing to commit all manner of wickedness and whoredoms. Then it says that Akish led his people away by their promise to do whatsoever thing he desired. In short, he administered secret combinations. To enter into a secret combination is the most abominable and wicked thing a man can do."

Burton locked onto Samuel and declared, "You've got this Oracle pegged. He fits that description and more. I don't know a whole lot about what you call secret . . . whatever . . . "

"Secret combinations: The oaths, the crime, the Mafia-type code of living."

"Yeah, well this Oracle is messing around with that kind of thing. Actually, I think, like you, that he really is playing footsie with the Devil and destroying lives in the process. There is one thing I really believe in, though I actually have no real . . . you know . . . I'm not really a religious person. But I do believe there is evil in the world, and there has to be something behind it making it happen —the same as I believe God is all good and powerful. You can't play with the Devil and win. Life doesn't work that way."

* * *

"He's gone, sir," the security man said to Reuben, then added, "His member name is Daniel."

"What do you mean, he's gone? How?"

The young man who had been promoted to chief gatekeeper stood before Reuben with a serious frown as he explained that during a routine check of personnel in the compound, they had come up one short among the sixty-four members that were accounted for each day. It was simple enough: Each commune rank-and-file member wore a wristband that was programmed to allow central security to monitor the whereabouts of each member any time it wished. The security program was usually run twice each day, morning and evening, to be sure that each commune member was present and accounted for. At a certain time each wristband was beeped, which required the wearer to press a button to answer the beep. In addition, an alarm would be sounded if a person ventured outside the perimeter of the compound. Similar bands were used all the time by the courts. In areas where prisons were jammed to the rafters, instead of giving convicted felons jail time, a judge might have a sensor device placed on the individual. And if the sentence called for that person to remain within a given radius—say an apartment—then if the felon strayed, the signal would alert authorities. Judges enjoyed slapping sensor bands on the ankles of felons who were not a danger to society in the usual sense of hardened criminals, but who certainly needed to be penalized all the same.

"Daniel" had not checked in electronically at the morning roll call. The system flashed a bright red light on the panel beside his name, indicating that he was not reporting in. Perhaps he was sleeping. The alarm did not indicate that he had left the compound, simply that he had failed to punch the button in response to the morning beep on his wristband. It was David who finally discovered the beeping sensory wrist mechanism cradled in a plastic Ziploc bag under warm running water in the basement utility room where Daniel stored his cleaning equipment each day after he had cleaned the rooms assigned to him. He had placed the sensor unit inside the bag after carefully cutting it from his wrist. The warm water was as close to human warmth as Daniel could manage. He had left the water running slowly through the night while he made his escape behind the limestone cliffs and walked to freedom.

It took him all night to walk and jog to Jackson Hole. Daniel had spent days planning his escape. He knew that by midmorning, at the very latest, they would detect he was missing. By that time he would be in Jackson Hole surrounded by tourists and able to blend in with the crowd. He wore a Dodger baseball cap that he had hoarded in his meager belongings. He had shaved all his hair below the cap to remove any sign of the bright carrot color that would be easy to spot on the streets of the resort town. His heavy, quilted jacket had a two-inch collar that he pulled up to touch the cap from behind. Except for the compound-issue, black quilted jacket that would be readily noticed by security, most everything else he was wearing would blend in with the crowd. He needed a different jacket.

It had been breakfast time at the Elk Café off the main route in Jackson Hole when Daniel slipped in, looked around, unobtrusively removed his black jacket, and, when the moment was right, traded it for a light brown ski jacket he found on the coat rack in the foyer where patrons hung their jackets and caps before being seated in the café. Out on the street once more, Daniel felt more secure in the neutral jacket. It was two sizes too large, but that didn't matter to Daniel. Actually, it was better. It made him look heavier and older, he thought.

The morning had been a long one, moving from store to store, from motel to hotel, up and down Jackson Hole in an effort to stay on the move. After making the phone call to Roy's place and leaving a message, Daniel kept on the move for the next six hours. He knew he needed a second plan if Roy was away, or if he chose not to return his call at the requested time. He had only five dollars left, all in quarters. He could not stand on the highway hitchhiking; Gateway security would spot him in seconds. His mind churned rapid-fire thoughts, trying to devise an alternate plan of action.

In his stress and confusion, Daniel felt that the last resort would be to turn himself in to the police and tell all that was happening in the compound. But he was afraid to do that. Rumor among the guys in the central kitchen at Gateway had it that certain higher-ups in the police department, as well as the sheriff's office, were paid by the Grand Oracle to return members of the order to the compound. Whether it was true or not, Daniel was not sure. He knew that he didn't want to test the accuracy of the rumor. Throughout the day he avoided all police.

\* \* \*

"You know what he looks like. So get out there and search!" Reuben sat hunched over the wheel, shaking his head in disgust as he watched his best-trained security boys fan out, moving with long strides along the sidewalk. They had to find that kid. Josiah wasn't going to take another security blunder well at all. And no one knew better than Reuben to what extreme the Oracle could carry his wrath.

Of course, the guards knew Daniel on sight, but they also knew that the skiing season was upon Jackson Hole in full force. It was the short week before Thanksgiving, and people took the week off. Boots and heavy ski jackets, mostly worn by the young and lively, crowded the streets. Searching like birds of prey for Daniel in this crowd was like trying to find someone at a rock concert.

But they had no choice. They had been commanded to find Daniel. That was all fine, but no one at security was certain that Daniel had come into Jackson Hole. He could have made contact with someone and been picked up outside the compound. Reuben didn't buy that. The kid would head for Jackson Hole and try to figure out an escape from that point. Reuben had a man at the commuter-size airport, another at the bus station, and watchers stationed along the highways in case Daniel decided to hitchhike. Sooner or later they would spot him. Reuben was sure of that.

Reuben was right. Daniel had just left the phone booth at the Chevron station on the corner of Pike and Commonwealth. It was noon, and Job, one of the more promising security men who had turned 21 last month, saw him and recognized the furtive look about the boy. Looking closer, he easily identified Daniel.

Job contacted compound control, asking for instructions as to apprehending the suspect. He looked down to clip his cell phone onto his belt. When he looked up, Daniel had slipped into the crowd that was standing three deep, waiting for the fleet of buses that pulled into the Pine Lodge Hotel. Job leaped from his blue Jeep and pushed bodies out of the way in an effort to catch sight of the light tan ski jacket. There were at least ten jackets of the same general color and look. It was hopeless. Job checked back with security control at the compound.

"At least we know he was in town at noon. We'll find the little creep," Reuben had said when he received word of the sighting. But two hours later the security men on the streets reported back that they had found nothing. It was then that Reuben began to fume. He wanted results. More important, the Grand Oracle insisted that Daniel be caught and disciplined.

Reuben himself roamed the several crowded streets of Jackson Hole. His security people had reported back at least fifteen times, giving the head of security an update every fifteen minutes. He kept crossing their paths as they scurried about the streets. It was getting dark. Light snow was beginning to fall across the frontier-like town, but the skiers who crowded the streets didn't seem to mind. In reality, they were thrilled with the coming storm—more snow meant more fun.

The fun would start for Reuben when he got hold of that slimy little redhead with big ideas. He would not be allowed to live; that was already a fact in Reuben's mind. Reuben wished he had Jeremiah out on the street to search for the young fugitive. Jeremiah was cloistered in the compound where Josiah and Reuben felt he was best needed—out of sight. The killing of that fellow in Provo was too fresh. They couldn't afford for Jeremiah to be pulled over by the police, even for a minor infraction of the law. His past was well documented, and his fingerprints would place him in federal prison with little more than a lightning-fast trial. A year ago he was wanted in a couple of Eastern states by two federal agencies for murder. Of course, that was last year. Since then, charred remains found in a Mississippi church bombing were tentatively identified by authorities as his body.

The identification was based on little evidence because the body was shattered by the bombing, and only fragments could be pieced together by the coroner. But from eyewitness reports and the fact that Jeremiah's van was parked several blocks from the bombing, they ruled that the body was that of the wanted criminal.

That was the week that Jeremiah came west at the request of Reuben, and with the Oracle's approval, joined Gateway. He took an immediate position as assistant to the chief of security. He and Reuben had been friends for the past ten years. Rarely did Jeremiah leave the compound; and even then he remained secluded in the cave, where he performed training tasks in fire power and explosives. He wore kidskin gloves most of the time. At other times he would spray a silicone solution that would seal across the grooves of his fingertips, creating a smooth, plastic-coated finish that lasted for hours to prevent leaving identifiable fingerprints. He had used the spray before following Roy. There were never fingerprints left behind when Jeremiah did a rare, outside-the-compound assignment for the Grand Oracle.

Reuben wished for Jeremiah. No one else possessed the cat-like instincts Jeremiah had perfected. Reuben dreaded the wrath of the Oracle that was surely coming. Two members in a short period of time trying to escape. The Oracle would not tolerate such lax security.

The white Jeep Grand Cherokee left the main road into downtown and veered to the right. Stephen was driving. Burton was in the passenger side of the front seat with a city map of Jackson Hole laid out on his lap. He had purchased it in Rexburg when they refueled at the Arco station.

"Now, when we get to the strip mall with the Albertsons store, I want you guys to let me out and keep circling the block. Go right one time and left the next; don't be too obvious. We don't know who is watching. The kid could be standing out there as bait, and we could fall into a trap," Burton cautioned.

"You don't really think it's a setup?" Stephen said.

"Naw, I don't. But we can't be too careful at this point. I want to scout the mall, and perhaps I can spot the kid. I have no idea what he looks like, but I have a built-in instinct for identifying people who are nervous and wary of strangers. Your usual tourist—and there are plenty around here as you can see—is very casual. He won't be."

When Stephen pulled away from the curb, Burton hopped over a puddle of slush. The weather had warmed up enough to melt the snow as it fell on the streets. He walked directly to the Albertsons store. There were many shoppers pulling into the parking lot, mostly four-wheel-drive vehicles crowding the fire lane. Thom stepped between two cars that had come to a halt to let a woman pushing a shopping cart pass. He kicked the slush from his shoes and looked around like any of the other dozen customers who were coming and going. He let his eyes roam the several store fronts adjacent to the supermarket, trying to discern the sort of person who was trying too hard to be casual.

Burton knew he would be young, somewhere in his early twenties. He had only the voice to go by, but in his mind the voice belonged to a young man who looked younger than his years. All he could visualize in his mind was a kid who looked like his mother had just combed his hair to go to church: fair skin, straight teeth, bright eyes, and a frightened look, suspicious of anyone who approached and spoke to him. After five minutes of glancing at strangers,

Burton's attention riveted on a young man who fit the age bracket. He noticed that the youth had passed by him twice. He stepped into the store and remained inside a couple of minutes.

* * *

"Report, security two. What's the status?" Reuben barked into the mouthpiece, wiping the heavy snowflakes from his eyebrows as he stood next to his vehicle across from the ski rental shop on Pine, where he had parked diagonally. Burton had been moving along the sidewalk when Reuben asked for a report from security two.

The crackling voice of security two had come through the unit. "I think I have a suspect who entered Albertsons three minutes ago. I'm standing at the far end of the parking lot. I have been by this store three times, so if I walk over there again, someone may notice I have a real curiosity about the place."

"To hell with that. Go into Albertsons and take a look at the suspect in the light. I'm on my way. I'll be in front of the market in two and a half minutes. If we have to, we'll take him bodily. We'll snag that little bastard. Do it now!"

Security two entered the electronically controlled entrance to Albertsons as Daniel exited at the other end of the store front. Security two moved rapidly up and down the several aisles but failed to spot the kid.

When Daniel emerged from the opposite set of electronic doors, he turned to his right and began slowly walking in front of the small shops that huddled next to Albertsons. Burton saw him and tracked him with his eyes. He noticed that the kid had not purchased groceries. Daniel's hands were shoved deep into the pockets of his tan ski jacket. Burton couldn't help noticing that the jacket was at least two sizes too large, but then kids nowadays like the baggy look. Convinced that this was the one he was searching for, Burton moved smartly along the covered sidewalk until he came up behind the kid. *Good grief! He could pass for fifteen,* Thom thought. After getting a side view of the clear, white, scrubbed cheeks, Thom spoke:

"Hey, do you happen to have the time?"

The boy's white face instantly faded whiter, and the freckles that covered his nose even lost some of their color. It was the look of a frightened puppy running in the middle of a freeway. He had his man.

" . . . Ah . . . ," Daniel stammered, "I don't have a watch. . . . Ah . . . I don't know."

"That's okay. It must be about seven, wouldn't you say?"

Daniel began to turn around when Burton said, "I'm Thom Burton, and I've come with Roy's friend Stephen from Provo to pick you up."

Daniel stood dead still and listened. Turning around slowly, he met Thom's eyes.

Thom smiled. "Yep, we're here. Right over there at the corner comes the Jeep. It's white and beautiful . . . and safe."

There appeared to be no sense of relief in the young man's expression. He was still stone cold, suspicious of Thom.

"You did ask for a ride, didn't you? If you're not expecting a white Jeep, then I'm sorry I bothered you. I thought you were someone else who called Roy this afternoon and asked for a ride from the Albertsons store."

Daniel stood a moment longer, studying Burton. Then, without a word, he broke into a run directly for the white Cherokee that was slowly entering the parking lot. Burton had already signaled to Stephen that he had their boy in tow.

Burton didn't try to figure out why the kid didn't verbally respond. He simply turned himself in the direction of the Cherokee and followed the kid at a brisk walk. The back door of the Cherokee swung open and the boy scrambled in, slamming it behind him. Thom reopened the door and climbed in beside the young man as Stephen took his foot off the brake pedal and slowly moved out of the parking lot behind a stream of cars.

Security two came out of the exit and failed to notice the white Jeep pull out of the parking lot and make a right turn. Snowflakes the size of quarters shrouded any vision beyond ten feet.

A Ford F-150 pickup, silver with chrome, came into the parking lot going the opposite direction. Daniel hit the floor. "That's one of them, the guy in the pickup. Don't let 'em see me. Please."

Burton glanced at the silver pickup and saw the driver's face. He also noticed the double lights on the roof of the cab. It was only a second that his attention riveted on the man and the pickup, but suddenly he knew he had seen that vehicle before. The guy inside was a mystery, but the new pickup looked oh, so familiar.

Stephen was halfway down the street when it struck Burton. It was a double-lamped cab roof that Burton remembered seeing when he had asked the guy in the pickup at the Double Tree if he was from Twin Falls. He had been evasive, not wanting to talk. Highly unusual, Burton recalled, for a person from Magic Valley not to be friendly. It had struck him as odd. Was that the same truck? If it was, why was it at the Double Tree the night Roy drove from Salt Lake to Provo and later died? Was there a connection?

"Stephen!" Burton shouted from the right side. "I'm getting out. I want to get a better look at that truck that passed us coming into the mall parking lot."

"What truck?"

"The one this kid here says was one of them."

"I didn't see it."

"Stop anyway. I'm going to hike back there. Go around the block a couple of times, and I'll meet you up there at the next intersection. I've got to get a look at that pickup and the guy in it."

Stephen didn't argue. He brought the Jeep to a sliding halt in the slush. Burton already had the door open and was stepping out. He loped toward the strip mall, snow hampering his vision. Along the snowbanked parking lot he watched like a wolf studying its prey as the silver pickup came back around and paused at the exit where Stephen had pulled out three minutes ago. Burton stood back, sheltered by a large pine and studied the Ford pickup as it idled ten feet from him. The license threw him. It was the characteristic bucking bronco plates of Wyoming. He had hoped it would be Idaho plates. Still, he studied the letters and numbers and put them to memory. He also decided to chance walking alongside the pickup to get a good view of the driver. He stepped from the shadow of the pine, and as he did so, the engine revved and the pickup pulled away. Burton stood looking as the pickup made its way onto the main street and disappeared. Damn. He knew it was the same kind of pickup. How many new Ford pickups have dual lights on the roof of the cab? He had never seen it before. But then maybe it was something new that was catching on.

He knew to not stand idly out in the open parking lot. He turned and raced up the street to the intersection and caught up with Stephen, who had just completed his first circling of the block.

Once free of the slow-moving local vehicles, Stephen put his foot to the pedal and moved more rapidly through the slushy street toward the main highway that would take the four of them to Idaho and on to Utah.

\* \* \*

The Oracle had named him Nathan for his size and long dark hair. Nathan filled the small office desk chair beyond its recommended weight limit. He weighed 273 pounds stripped. But it was not his size that gave him an edge over the other youths at Gateway. It was his aptitude for electronics and computers. He had come into the compound two years before, and Gateway had become a home that he loved. It mattered little to Nathan that he was never allowed beyond the main gate. He, like Jeremiah, who worked in the communications center with him, found fulfillment in the vast reaches of the Net, the fax, and the sophisticated surveillance system they had created.

Nathan had cleared a close security screening that the Oracle devised for all ten of the Gateway security people—nine males and one female. They guarded the front gate, kept all members from the cave, and were generally responsible for law and order in the compound. They bowed to the demands of three people: the Oracle, Reuben, and Jeremiah. All others at Gateway answered to them.

Nathan had the run of the compound. Lately, his only distraction was the new inductee with the dark hair—Rachel. He knew from the computer files that her true name was Brenda, that she came from the Bay Area, had been a student at Redlands. He had made it his business to learn all the details about Brenda. He liked her. He also knew that she was a ward of Mother Martha; that meant mind-altering drugs and a myriad of other mind-twisting methods to create a subservient young woman. Nathan knew he could do nothing to stop the indoctrination. However, even Mother Martha had lamented how she hated to subject such a lovely creature to her program. Nathan continued to dream of Brenda, who was in her room not twenty yards from him. His thoughts delighted him, but he knew that if he allowed himself to indulge too much in fantasies of a beautiful girl, it would hamper his effectiveness at Gateway. He limited his daydreaming.

Nathan seldom took a shift at the main gate; Jeremiah saw to that. He was needed in the communications room. Nathan willingly spent fifteen hours a day inside the cave in the communications center. He never asked questions. The Oracle had bragged to Reuben about what a loyal subject he had in Nathan, ignoring the fact that it was Reuben who had recruited Nathan when the young giant had gone AWOL from the Coast Guard in New Jersey. He had welcomed the security of Gateway to wait out the years until he would be free to resume some sort of life on the outside once again. They had never found it necessary to indoctrinate Nathan with drug therapy. He came obedient and ready to serve a master. It puzzled Jeremiah how a man so intelligent could be so subservient to the Oracle. Jeremiah was himself anything but subservient. He obeyed, but it was because he had made a decision to do so based on commissions and possible freedom one day. He enjoyed fantasizing about how he would bolt and resettle in Latin America. Nathan, on the other hand, had no future plans that Jeremiah could discern.

"I picked up some action on the police band last night," Nathan said casually to Jeremiah. "I can't say for sure, but some police dispatcher in Jackson seemed pretty frustrated with one of the units who radioed in about a white Cherokee picking up some subject. I don't know if it had anything to do with the escape of that kid Daniel. Should I report it to Reuben?" he asked.

Jeremiah went on sipping coffee and surfing the Net for a few minutes.

Finally he answered. "It's up to you. But if you were going to tell Reuben, you should have informed him last night."

"I tried. He was not at any of the usual phones. But I'm asking you, should I tell him now?"

"Nope." Jeremiah shrugged. "It's probably too late to do anything about it. If it comes up, tell him you tried to alert him, but he was out of contact. No big deal."

\* \* \*

"Sheriff Harmon here, Mr. Massey. We've had some action here in Jackson concerning some of the people from Gateway that may or may not be significant."

Though it was long past normal working hours, Massey was still in his office taking calls from FBI agents in Walnut Creek. One of the fashionable malls in the Bay Area had received a bomb threat. The story had been unfolding throughout the day and into early evening. It was completely unrelated to Gateway or anything happening in Jackson Hole, but it required Massey's attention as local law enforcement in Contra Costa County investigated a possible terrorist group emerging. When the call came in from the sheriff in Jackson, Massey shifted his attention from the bomb scare to a possible break in the situation at Gateway.

"What's going on, sheriff?"

"We're keeping a low profile, but one of the local police officers forgot and used his radio to report that a couple of pickups from Gateway had been circling the downtown streets for a while. The dispatcher reminded him to get off the radio and use a pay phone. When the officer called back, he said he first saw one of the Gateway vehicles in Jackson two hours ago. The driver didn't seem to be doing anything unusual except that the only time he got out of his vehicle was to fill up with gas. He had been circling town for the whole time. Then a few minutes ago another unit reported some action at a strip mall not far from the center of town. Apparently, one of the guys from Gateway parked his vehicle and walked into the Albertsons supermarket. He was in there for a while and came out without having purchased anything visible. The cop on duty watched him the whole time. He said the guy just moved around the store; then he came out looking in all directions. It appeared to the officer that he was searching for someone. While the man was inside the store, the other officer, who stayed with the car, reported watching a young man who seemed to be in a confused state walking in the shadows near the store. Suddenly, the kid dashed through the corner of the parking lot and got into a white car."

"What model of white car?"

"The officer wasn't sure, with visibility so short, but it looked like some type of 4X4. He can't be certain."

"Are you thinking what I am, sheriff?"

"Do you think the young fellow at the mall has escaped from Gateway and the boys are out tracking him down?"

"That's what I think is happening. What about sending out an all-points alert? You have authority to go statewide and farther. Do you want to issue an all-points for a white 4X4?"

"I don't know how much good that would do. Do you have any idea how many white 4X4s there are around here?"

"Well, stay on it. I'll be here in my office until midnight. Call me if you hear anything more. If it's later, you have my home number. Keep me up to date on this one. It may be the break we were hoping for."

"Right. I'll do that."

# Chapter 15

As they traveled slowly over the crest, the large snowflakes belted the car with winds up to fifty miles per hour. Stephen remained steady at the wheel while Burton questioned Daniel. It got him nowhere. The trauma of escaping, trying to avoid being found, only to be sighted by Reuben's security force on the streets of Jackson, and desperately eluding them again had taken its toll on Daniel. The young man was close to a catatonic state, frozen in silence. Still Burton persisted.

Samuel finally leaned over and cautioned Thom about probing too hard too soon. "He needs professional help. Surely there are doctors who specialize in helping people who have been traumatized."

Burton thought about that for a few moments, then reached for the cell phone and asked information for the Barkley Television Network in Oakland. He got the number and placed the call, letting the phone ring insistently. It was nearly eight-thirty in Oakland. Who would still be in at this hour? A recorded voice gave the hours the offices were open, then advised that if the caller had news of a breaking story to call the station number. The number followed. Burton punched it in.

He held his hand over the receiver as he spoke to the group in the Jeep. "I'm trying to reach a journalist I met while we were on the Gateway tour." The news station apparently remained open all night, but it took the next ten minutes and twenty dollars in telephone charges to reach Morris Turnbull, who was a self-styled authority on cults. Burton finally got through to him at his condo in Berkeley.

Morris remembered Burton, so Burton cut right to the core of the situation. "Hey, man, we need help." He explained the whole situation: Roy's death, the call from Daniel, his fear of revealing anything about the compound, and Stephen's concern for his daughter. He brought Morris all the way to the present—the four of them trucking along in heavier snow than Stephen had ever driven in. He had the Cherokee in four-wheel drive as he listened to Burton rehearse the entire series of events.

Having brought his associate up to date, Burton listened to Morris explain that the kid probably needed the help of a doctor he knew in New Mexico. "Do you want me to call her? I did an interview with her two months ago. You might be interested in what she has to say. I'll fax you the article if you'll tell me where."

"Good idea. Would you please call her? Tell her we can bring Daniel down if she can see him immediately."

"Tell him I'll pay all costs," Samuel said from the front seat as he glanced over at young Daniel.

"Did you hear that?"

Morris had heard the voice in the background. He agreed to try to set up an appointment with the doctor. The two hung up, but not before Morris wished Burton good luck finding a seat on any plane from Salt Lake to Albuquerque; that is, if Dr. Mucranski had time to see the young man. Morris assured Burton that he would buzz him back as soon as he got word from the doctor. His call came fifteen minutes later as the Jeep was pulling into the same Arco station they had stopped at earlier in the evening.

Stephen filled up the tank, pulled sandwiches and a jug of hot chocolate out of the back of the Jeep, handing them to Samuel to distribute, and got back into the warm Cherokee when the phone buzzed. In clipped tones Morris assured Burton that the doctor would see the boy if he could get down there tomorrow.

All the way from Blackfoot to Pocatello, Idaho, to the south, Burton called around for reservations. None. Samuel took the cell phone and began asking information about private charters out of Provo or Salt Lake. Their offices were closed, of course. He moved his calling north to Ogden. He had luck: Ken Roberts, who operated a charter jet and two freight helicopters, happened to be in his hangar when Samuel got through.

"It'll be kinda pricey for me to drop everything in the morning, fly down to Provo to pick up your friends, and fly them to New Mexico."

"Can you do it?"

"Oh, sure. I'm just warning you that it won't come cheap."

Samuel didn't ask how much. He knew he had a quarter-million-dollar limit on his gold American Express card. He simply gave Roberts the card number so he could check out the limit and told him he would expect the small

Lear jet to be on the ground, ready to pick up Burton and a companion, by seven-thirty in the morning. It was tempting for Samuel to accompany the two, but he had already called Katherine and asked her to make reservations on whatever flight she could get out of Salt Lake City to his hometown of Boise, on Thanksgiving Day.

* * *

The Oracle had sent for Martha shortly after learning of Daniel's escape. He wanted an explanation of why, after all the indoctrination and the assurances Martha had given him, he had still lost two members in a week.

"They are resisting your methods. Why? What is happening that two can become so determined to leave the compound and escape? Martha, I do not blame you for their escape; their escape is a flaw in security. I lay at your feet, however, the desire that seems to have welled up within them to want to leave us."

Martha stood by the floor-to-ceiling windows that looked out on the enclosed patio with an empty fountain in the center. Two robins were perched on the ceramic edge of the fountain's desolate pool. They must have come down from Canada to escape the harshness of winter. They were on their way south to enjoy the sunshine. Martha longed to go with them. Anywhere would have been preferable to this very office where she was required to defend her science-of-mind alteration. She slowly turned to meet the eyes of the Oracle. She locked onto his tiny pupils and answered his question. "Not all humans respond in the same manner to stimuli. Any scientist will tell you that in any sampling there are dynamics of uniqueness. I have no answer as to why two young men would want to leave here, not after undergoing the kind of reorientation I gave them. You have told me who they are, and I know of no reason why those two did not remain loyal. I assure you they did not manifest any rebellious spirit while undergoing indoctrination."

Martha spoke precisely and without fear of any sort. Her very thin lips matched the narrowness of her eyes. She may have been beautiful at one time, in a severe way. She was like an aging European model in form, with a sad countenance. She had come into the order as a specialist and had worked long hours to achieve what she considered excellent results. Her qualifications were impressive. She had the best training available—not even the CIA had better instructors than she.

The Oracle stood seething beside his desk. He was prone to make quick responses. His anger with security had abated somewhat, but it returned when Martha came into his office. When he did not respond to Martha's defense of the science of mind alteration, she added, "You surely know that this sort of brain manipulation is not an exact science. After all, we have had only the latter part of this century to experiment with the mind. At least in the western world . . ."

"Silence!" the Oracle commanded. "I don't want to hear any more of your theories. When you came here, or should I say when I dredged you up from that lab in New York, you told me that you had been instructed by the masters in South America. You told me . . . "

"I told you that it was not possible to alter all minds." She was impervious to his brand of madness. She had seen too many others in her work to ever bow to his demands. Not any more. This tactless frontal assault on her skill would vanish from her mind like a fog in the morning sun, "I remember you asking me what percentage of young people could be indoctrinated to your set of standards of conduct. I remember clearly informing you that it would never be a hundred percent. And you said that you could take care of the few who refused to change."

"Don't remind me of what I said," the Oracle shouted as he paced in front of his desk. He paused, then in a quieter tone he continued. "I recall asking you if you could detect in the indoctrination stages whether a particular person would fail to respond to the therapy. You assured me that you could."

Martha moved back to the window. She noticed that the robins had fled. "I was wrong." There was a rising edge to her voice as she spoke to the window. "Do you have anything else to discuss with me?" Irritation punctuated the tone of her voice. With that statement she moved toward the door. Her fingers were beginning to tremble. She knew she was very much under the thumb of this religious leader, and that he had the power to take care of her and anyone else who crossed him. She now knew there was no longer any choice. She had to leave Gateway, and she needed to make her move soon. She stopped at the door and waited for a response to her leaving. It didn't come. He said nothing as she stood poised to walk out of the office and return to the cave.

She should have told the Oracle straight out about Rachel—another resister. Brenda, or Rachel as she was known in Gateway, would never tolerate this insane incarceration. She was a free spirit. But Martha no longer cared to inform the Oracle of anything. He had lost all the attraction she had once felt toward him, and he no longer meant anything to her. Like the robins, she was going to escape. The question was how.

"I do have one other thing to discuss with you." The Oracle had altered his tone of voice from anger to a near-normal conversational intonation. He could switch from heated emotion to ice, then to glad-hander in seconds.

Martha had hoped he would not detain her. She had listened to all she cared to. What now?

"I have a certain group of Asian surgeons coming in the next two weeks; there will be a team of three. I would hope that you will treat them with the utmost respect. They will not be seen by anyone but security. They will be housed in the dorm inside the cave. I suggest you learn from these eminent men of science."

Martha's curiosity captured her better judgment. She asked the question, "And what makes these surgeons so special?" She remembered Jeremiah telling her the surgeons were coming to Gateway.

The Oracle had not planned to tell Martha of his arrangements to use a program of cloning. The less said to anyone in the compound the better. "It might be best if you know very little about what this medical team has in mind."

"Fine."

She pushed open the office door, set to exit, when she heard his quiet, eerie voice say, "No, on the contrary, I think you should know. You will learn about it soon enough when these surgeons do what they will be paid to do. Close the door and sit down."

Martha did as she was told. She wished she had remained silent and not asked about the surgeons. She wanted to be on her way down the hall of the executive wing and back to the cave. In reality, she knew she longed more than ever to be out of his sight . . . forever. She sat uncomfortably awaiting what he had to tell her.

He was deliberately silent for long enough to make Martha wonder if she were to be involved in some technical way with the surgical team. Then he spoke. "Surely, you have been aware of what has been happening over the last year or so with cloning techniques. Do you recall hearing about Dolly, the sheep that Ian Wilmut made with his cloning experiment at the Roslin Institute in Edinburgh, Scotland? He did some genetic engineering and cloned a sheep in the exact image of another. He did it by perfecting the Hill-Barstomere separation." There was a smugness, an intellectually condescending tone as he spoke to Martha. He telegraphed to her that he had superior knowledge of human engineering process and could not help sharing bits of it with her, a lowly human, whose training would soon become outdated.

"What do you want of me?"

"Oh, nothing. I simply thought it would be wise on my part to forewarn you that I intend to take your recommendation and use that young lady you are now programming—Rachel—and clone her."

She listened, but failed to have any emotional response. She knew enough about cloning, having read tomes of it on the Internet. She knew that to take tissue from Rachel would not be harmful. The girl would never know she had been cloned if they chose not to disclose the information to her, and if they used a surrogate mother.

"Dr. Chang has a select group of oriental women who, by the way, are more than willing to be surrogate mothers during the cloning process. I may not have told you, but I plan to use my tiny island off Mexico to do the experiments. We'll begin the process with your Rachel. Mexico has taken no steps to prevent cloning; besides, how will they know? I want to raise up a generation of clones in my lifetime, male and female. In the process I intend to alter their minds through genetic alterations. Then do you know what I plan to do?"

Martha stared at the Oracle, focusing her eyes on his narrow chin, as little shivers coursed up her spine and a palpable shudder went through her body. This entire scheme of things was becoming too weird, too involved in mind and body control even for Martha. She reasoned that what she did could be undone; not so with surgery. How she wished she were safely ensconced in some other country. She studied the Oracle with weary eyes. His arrogance and by-passing rules of conduct were strangely becoming repulsive to her, but she knew she had to suppress her venom toward him or be taken out immediately. Still, she could not resist one comment. "Will you clone yourself?"

His eyes narrowed and his chin withdrew. He did not respond to her question. Yet, she knew that one of the clones would be a carbon copy of this evil man. Not surprising.

The Oracle continued with his train of thought. "This same team of doctors, and this ought to interest you immensely, are in the forefront of robotic implantation. I know that you understand the process of implanting chips in the brains of animals; we've talked about this. With proper placement one can manipulate mental and physical actions. They have already shown it is possible in Japan with cats and dogs. They have a chip so small that they can implant it in a roach. Amazing, isn't it?" Josiah threw back his head and laughed as if he had thought of a very funny story. Martha remained stone silent.

"You ought to learn all you can about these implants. Let me tell you, our present method of programming is labor intensive. I plan to change all of that. I intend to create humans who are alike and can be programmed to do as I wish."

She studied the man a moment longer, then said, "It's playing God."

"Exactly. And you are not with your drug-oriented method? Come, come, Martha, you have been playing God with the minds of these young people since they have arrived here, and others long before that. So what? Let others fight over the ethical, legal, and social implications of applied cloning and chip manipulation. What is that to me? While they debate and pass international laws to protect the human race, I will have near-perfect people to welcome my God to this earth. Oh, my dear, you will see. These doctors are very special."

Her limbs were jelly. She had seen so much, been so involved in one experiment after another. She, of course, had manipulated hundreds of other humans, yet somehow this man and his motives were different. Why did the Oracle's plans affect her in this way? This was simply another step up the ladder of human manipulation. Yet somehow it struck her as morally wrong.

A look of disbelief registered on her face. The Oracle could see that Martha was physically shaken by his latest revelation. That was okay by him. He would not need her much longer, not when the surgical team got through.

\* \* \*

Dr. Andrea Mucranski was currently a research fellow at the University of New Mexico at Albuquerque. The honey-blond Hungarian psychologist smiled briefly and nodded to Burton as he stepped into the stark-white examining room at the Farwell Institute. Dr. Mucranski had been one of the chief architects in the design of the facility. She was a native of Hungary, born in Budapest a year after the first anti-Communist uprising in 1956. She was a pampered product of the Communist society in that country in former days. Educated in the public schools, she grew up in the Communist Party with her parents, who were loyal to the party. Her scholastic abilities enabled her to receive a full scholarship to the University of Budapest, from her freshman year to the completion of her Ph.D. in clinical psychology and her specialty of behavior modification.

Disillusioned with the Communist Party, Dr. Mucranski had hoped for an uprising that would overthrow the government, which was under the thumb of the Soviet Union. It came, but she had already taken matters into her own hands: She had escaped to Austria five years prior to the downfall of the Eastern Bloc nations. While working in Austria, she was offered a position at the University of New Mexico in the United States and became a part-time psychologist at the Farwell Institute, with special duties in deprogramming the brainwashed at the mental health facility. She had seen much trauma when she visited Moscow's Sverdlovsk Institute for the mentally disturbed. The old Soviet Union had destroyed many human minds before its demise.

Dr. Mucranski lately had devoted an inordinate amount of her time to deprogramming young people who had been mentally damaged by cults they had joined. Families sought her help for their college-age children who, in one way or another, had fallen under the influence of leaders of cults, not all of which were in America. She had patients from several countries.

"Have you heard of the Gateway cult in Wyoming, under the iron thumb of one Grand Oracle Josiah?" Burton asked her when they settled into a discussion of Daniel, who had been taken to his room.

"Yes, I know of him. I was told by your friend when he called that the young man you brought with you has been living at the compound in Wyoming."

"It's really great of you to take him on such short notice, Dr. Mucranski." Burton then explained to her that his associate, Samuel Meyers, would pay all expenses incurred to deprogram Daniel. "It is good of you to devote your time to this stressed-out kid."

"That is quite all right. I love my work and hope to help this Daniel. I'm very much open to helping these kids that are pulled from the pit that these self-styled prophets drop them into. Do you realize this Daniel is a very bright young man? If I were to guess, I would say that all the young people under the Oracle's control are very bright. I think Daniel will yet do well in life. I am sure of it. Of course, the scars will remain, but don't all of us have a few scars in life?"

Thom Burton liked this very practical woman of real intellect. She spoke so positively. But he wanted answers, so he said, "What we are interested in immediately is the state of this young man's mind and what he knows about what is going on at the compound. We were reluctant to probe him too much for fear it would cause further damage to his already programmed mind." Thom didn't reveal how hard he had tried to grill the kid—all the way from Jackson Hole to Rexburg.

"You were wise not to do further damage by questioning him," she commented. "The young man needs rest and a rebuilding of his self-esteem. However, he has already spoken to me of some of his experiences in the compound. I told him I would be talking to you about those experiences. I must caution you, however, that he is not ready to speak to you or to any authorities in law enforcement until I give consent. I hope I am clear in this matter."

Burton sensed that the petite female doctor had a steel rod for a backbone. In Eastern Europe, before she escaped, she must have experienced some difficult circumstances. She obviously was a strong and forthright person. According to Morris, she was the best.

"I've had very little experience with cult groups," Burton volunteered. He and Dr. Mucranski had gone to the cafeteria for coffee. Burton sat on a bench across the long table from the doctor. They talked of a possible special program he would develop featuring her work with the psychologically injured. He told her that when things settled down, he would convince his boss to come in at a different angle than Morris had taken with his special report. Burton thought it could be worked into a full-blown, one-hour special on the Institute and the sort of problems the doctor had to deal with. It would be hot.

Thom had been in touch with his boss the day before and explained everything that had transpired. Healy, the boss, was immediately concerned. "Burton, I'm warning you. A crazy like your Josiah can flip, and you may end up coming home on a flight in a special cargo hold for coffins. Do you read me?" Burton had laughed it off.

Thom knew that he didn't fear encounters in life like most people. When he was a boy, he would come home from sports activities with scrapes and broken limbs. His mother would shake her head and declare that it would be okay to fear a few things in life. Strange, but even considering Roy's death and

Daniel's plea for help, Josiah in all his pomp had not made a direct impact on Burton's own underdeveloped sense of fear.

The next time they met, Dr. Mucranski spent a good twenty minutes explaining what she had learned from Daniel during the past two days. She had carefully led him along as he felt like discussing why he had run away from the compound, but she had asked no direct questions that would upset him. She was able to learn that Daniel was afraid that he was going to be killed by the Grand Oracle or his chief of security. He kept repeating his fears of the Oracle as he moved in and out of a variety of subjects, such as his youth.

Growing up in St. Louis with a lawyer father and a devoted mother came into the picture. He spoke of pets, plays, movies, and neighborhood games, plus his first encounter with girls, his life on campus at Missouri State, his love of literature, and his enjoyment of his graduate work. He divulged that he was still eighteen when he received his BA degree. A genius! At intervals Daniel would revert to the compound and his deathly fear of the Oracle, who once made him enter a semi-dark, soundless room at the extreme end of the cave where missile-launching military hardware was stored. He saw it.

Daniel had broken down then and voluntarily told the Hungarian doctor about his best friend, Seth. He had wept openly, his words coming in a rush. "They executed him for leaving the compound. He was on his way to talk to the sheriff. He told me he was going. He was going to tell the sheriff about the cave and the illegal . . . They caught him . . . and in a terrible ceremony . . . they broke his neck. They made it look like an accident in a jeep." The boy cried silently for several minutes, his whole body shaking with emotion. " . . . I . . . I was at the execution. I saw his body on a flat board; he was ghostly white. It all happened in the cave. They have rooms in the cave. They have a worship room where the Oracle comes in wearing a red robe."

The doctor related that once his emotions had been tapped, Daniel went on in this manner, speaking only to Dr. Mucranski. Repeatedly he dissolved into tears and, like a perpetual CD, repeated verbatim all that he had witnessed, over and over again. At last, with her commanding voice, Dr. Mucranski silenced Daniel, then injected a medication that relaxed his muscles and put him to sleep.

When she told Burton all Daniel had said, Thom was confident that every word the kid had uttered was exactly the way it had happened at the compound.

He had heard a lot of stories of horror in his experience as a journalist, but nothing as graphic as Daniel's sad tale. He spent the next half-hour with Dr. Mucranski, comparing his notes with hers.

"You need to know one other thing about what may be happening at Gateway."

"What's that?"

"When I examined Daniel this morning, I had a hunch. I inspected the flesh between his toes. There are needle marks. So I looked more carefully between the creases and among the hair of his underarms. There are needle marks there as well."

"Drugs."

"I'm afraid so."

"I warn you again," she said sternly, "no one is to interview this young man until I say so. I have full rights in this matter. You understand, I hope. His mental stability is at stake. I also beg you not to go to the authorities yet. There is time. I need a week or more before news of this gets out—I want your word on this. The only reason I related all that he has told me is due to your genuine and devoted interest in his welfare. I feel that you have a compassionate spirit about you and that you are deeply concerned with his future. Otherwise, you would not have gone to such lengths to get him to me." The doctor smiled. "I know all this is hard to grasp at first. But I must have your word that you will not go to the authorities quite yet."

Burton knew the authorities had a right to be informed, but he tended to play both sides of the street when it came to an exclusive story. "Sure, sure . . . anything you say," he promised.

"Perhaps it would help you to know a little background information about the Oracle Josiah. I was reviewing it only this morning. Why don't you come to my office and I'll pull up his file."

Dr. Mucranski led Thom into her small, dark office on the second floor of the Institute. He looked around at the organized mess inherent to research. A PC dominated the center wall cabinet behind her desk, which was piled with papers and books clipped open at specific passages. On both sides of her computer center were large bookcases filled with a variety of books, mostly textbooks related to her field. Stacked haphazardly on the floor beside the desk were over two dozen books on cults of the world.

"Have a seat, Mr. Burton." Dr. Mucranski turned the wand on the side of her vertical blinds to let in a faint light. She sat down behind her desk. Being a small woman, her adjustable desk chair had been raised as high as possible to elevate her to a comfortable working position at her desk.

"So you know the Oracle?" Thom inquired.

"Yes. That is, I have never met him personally, but I have done my homework. I know who he is. So do government agencies that at times have to deal with these communal groups. I know because they have come to me for background information. I have a small staff, mostly graduate students, who have done an admirable job of collecting information about cults currently functioning in this country and throughout the world. We have done a full study of this person who titles himself The Grand Oracle Josiah."

"Will you let me look at his file?" Burton could hardly sit quietly in the plastic, body-formed chair in front of the doctor's desk, now aware that she had done a thorough study of the man.

"Yes, I'll share some of our findings with you, but first you must understand what the man is attempting to achieve in this center he has created. Above all, remember you are dealing with a mind that has been shaped by an environment of wealth and isolation. I'll explain in a moment. First, let's talk about the type of young people he targets, personalities who are vulnerable to the enticement of his propaganda.

"Many young people like Daniel downstairs see the world as hostile, often unjust. If you look at the American society, you will see the divorce rate now at seventy percent and violent crime out of control. Add to that the growing paralysis of our—pardon me—*your* government, with each political party doing its best to thwart the efforts of the other in curbing these social ills. Life often becomes threatening and illogical to sensitive, intelligent, young people like Daniel. Many have tried to find answers through traditional, mainline, religious affiliation. Unfortunately, many of these churches seem to have a collective death wish and have left the domain of religion and embarked upon a course of social gospel actions, such as providing an unrealistic view of life as it really is. This policy has spiritually disemboweled them."

Dr. Mucranski turned around in her swivel chair and placed her hands on the keyboard of her computer. She continued to speak to Burton with her back to him as the PC booted itself. "There is no question that America has a social and spiritual sickness. The inability of governmental, religious, and private institutions to deal with the breakdown of society or with some of the aggressive actions of individuals and organizations has resulted in the rise of Utopian societies. I had another young person in here. He said he had been at Gateway for a short while; somehow he got away and ended up here. I seem to be the referral for these types. Anyway, he left here after a week and refused to make any statements, contact the authorities, or anything of that nature. Just left. I have no idea where he ended up. I have no proof of what he told me, but if half of what he said is true, then this Oracle is bad news. That poor young man who took off stilll needed my help. If they ever break up that group, I will be busy for the next year trying to rehabilitate some of those young people.

"You see, when people are confused to the point that they feel they can no longer cope in society as it is—sheer reality—they sometimes move toward separation and seclusion, blocking out that which they cannot deal with. Our friend Josiah is one of those who feels he has seen the breakdown of society. Not only does he want to separate himself, but he desires to pull others out of a sick and wicked world along with him. He feels that he can create a better . . . no, change that . . . He is convinced that he can create a *perfect* world through mind manipulation of young people who will then correct the future of man. The Oracle has been effective for several years in ferreting out young people who are susceptible to his brand of cult indoctrination."

The computer monitor displayed a long list of file directories. Dr. Mucranski opened one labeled Oracle. Subdirectories appeared. The information on the Oracle had been carefully organized by subject matter. The doctor selected a file named Profile and pulled up an extensive biographical characterization of the Oracle.

"I'll scan through this and give you the highlights of this man. He comes from a wealthy family. I'm sure you have read about the DeWitts of Maryland: The grandfather made a fortune in shipping. Then Josiah's father increased that during World War II when he supported all sides in transporting goods and contraband.

"Josiah was raised on an estate in Maryland. He was never allowed to mix socially with young people that his parents disapproved of, and they were very selective. His social development was limited. He attended neither public nor private schools. His education came from carefully screened tutors. One of his tutors was steeped in the philosophy of Nietzsche, the famous German philosopher. Nietzsche believed, as did Hitler, that a super race of human beings was possible. Josiah was taught that throughout history certain superior individuals were created to be beacons or leaders to the world, such as Alexander the Great, Napoleon and others, and that society in the era when one of those superhumans lived ought to support and follow him. Josiah came to the conclusion that he was one of these special human beings destined to alter the course of mankind."

Dr. Mucranski tapped keys to scroll down the screen. Burton had moved his chair to the side of her desk so he could see the screen as well. "It has only been in the last several years that he has surfaced as a cult leader. Apparently, he had to wait until the death of his father. . . . By the way, his father died a rather mysterious death on his estate in Maryland. A full investigation by the local police turned up nothing except that he had somehow died from suffocation while he was alone in his quarters on the estate. No real evidence was found of foul play, and all the principal people in his life provided witnesses of their whereabouts at the time of death.

"Josiah DeWitt's mother had died some years before, and he was an only child. When he gained complete control of the family fortune a few months after the death of his father, he began construction on his so-called Gateway. His family had owned the property in Jackson Hole for decades and often vacationed there in their private, secluded lodge. Josiah removed the family lodge and constructed at enormous cost—upwards of one-hundred-million dollars—the compound as it now stands."

Dr. Mucranski turned to Burton and asked, "Didn't you say you have seen the layout?"

"Yes. I toured it with some of my associates. This guy has used the latest technology throughout. I was impressed with that part of the commune."

"I agree. Of all the cults I have personally visited or viewed on film, his is the most elaborate, and the environment is the most controlled. One large, main structure houses all aspects of living and working. To me it looked like a well-appointed retirement center, only much more. Did you see the Oracle's private swimming pool?"

"No, we were not allowed to visit certain areas of the compound, including the residential wings of the building."

"They say he has purified water delivered by a service weekly. They drain the pool and refill it with purified drinking water—very expensive. But it also reveals the meticulous nature of the man. He eats no meat, is fit, and as far as we have been able to determine he has no vices. He doesn't seem to be using any of the young people for his own personal desires. I'm not sure he has the usual passions of man. His passion is his cause, his dream."

"What is his dream?"

"Oh, he intends to create a super race of young people, programmed to do no wrong. He will remove choice from the lives of those who will be part of his new world. Free will, with his latest methods, will no longer be part of human behavior. You see, from reports I have, he believes God has designated him to act as his special oracle, charged with correcting the irregular nature of man on earth. Through total obedience to the will of the Oracle, mankind can function in a perfect state of bliss. It's a kind of Garden of Eden concept where total innocence prevails—no good or evil—simply bliss for all."

Burton listened intently, then asked, "How is he able to achieve this state of innocence with his people?"

"He has devised a carefully structured retraining program—a combination of drugs and psychological indoctrination. At the conclusion of the mind training young people appear satisfied with their docile role. They function at the compound in a variety of assignments without any apparent spirit of rebellion. I do not know exactly what his formula is for maintaining such a level of success with his subjects. However, the fact that Daniel ran away, and that the young man Seth was killed—according to Daniel—because he was going to go to the police, would indicate that the Oracle's reprogramming success rate is short of one hundred percent."

"That's right," Burton said. "Some must rebel. Look at Daniel; he escaped."

"Of course. Daniel was apparently able to maintain some of his former free spirit. It didn't take as effectively with him as it may have with others up there. I would guess there are others whose desire for freedom will drive them to resist being totally dominated. Daniel is the second I have seen from the compound in Wyoming."

# Chapter 16

The time was seven in the evening when Stephen spoke on the phone with Burton. Anney stood leaning against the door jamb, listening to the conversation. She detected from Stephen's response that the young man, Daniel, had suffered at the hands of the compound people. She studied Stephen's mouth repeating some of the things that were being spoken and asking questions about drugs, indoctrination, and discipline.

"Mr. Thorn, or rather Stephen, where did you say your daughter attended school? Didn't you mention in the car that she had disappeared from Redlands?"

"Yeah, why?"

"Interesting . . . "

Burton's pause annoyed Stephen. "Why?" he repeated.

"Well, from what this Daniel has told the doctor here, he was a student at Redlands as well, doing a brief study."

"Are you telling me that there may be a connection between our Brenda and this Daniel, or with that cult group in Wyoming? Is that what you're saying?" Stephen's voice sped up. He wanted an answer, an answer from Burton.

"I'm just saying that your daughter and Daniel came from the same school. Let me tell you what I'm going to do. I think I can get in touch with the school authorities and determine just who Daniel is. He hasn't told us much about his family, but we are piecing it together. He has to be certain he can trust us before he will give out that kind of information. I can find out by tomorrow. I'm contacting the school and I'll get to the core of this whole thing.".

Anney listened. She could not hear all that was being discussed, but she did hear that Brenda was part of the phone discussion. She reached out, grabbing Stephen's shoulder as he sat on the edge of the bed. Anything concerning Brenda was intensely important to Anney.

"Stephen, what does Brenda have to do with this thing that has happened in Wyoming?"

Stephen was trying desperately to hear every word from Burton and at first ignored Anney.

She was too insistent."Stephen!" she shouted.

Stephen soon hung up, then turned to explain to Anney all that Burton had said.

"Are they doing to Brenda the same thing they have done to that poor kid down in New Mexico? They drugged him, didn't they?" Anney began moving her head from side to side in a mother's total despair.

"Anney! Listen to me. We don't know that Brenda is in that compound." Like Anney, he felt that she was, though there was no proof. Stephen wanted to soften the impact of his conversation with Burton. He wished Anney had not been in the room. This latest information about the condition of Daniel he knew would go down hard with Anney. It was hard enough for him to hear Burton tell what Dr. Mucranski had surmised had happened to Daniel at Gateway. It boiled down to mind-altering drugs and physical deprivation.

"Yes," Stephen uttered, placing both hands behind his neck and dropping his head. He felt so helpless. As a father, what could he do? He felt so strapped for a logical answer to free her. "The medical doctor in charge of the institute down there told Burton that Daniel had been subjected to some complex indoctrination and . . . '' Stephen pressed his fingers tightly to the back of his neck and squeezed his arms together in frustration, "Oh, I can't believe all of this. She says that Daniel is still in shock and it will take a few days for her to make a complete evaluation of his condition, but hopefully he will recover."

"I knew it," Anney responded, turning her head to the wall. Tears began cascading down her cheeks. Her world was crumbling. "Brenda, oh, Brenda," she whispered to the wall in utter frustration.

Stephen dropped his hands from behind his head, stood up, and walked over to Anney. He pulled her away from the wall and held her close. She burrowed her head into his chest and wept openly. He could not resist the tears forming in his own eyes. It was all so unreal, so much shocking and horrifying news from hell that both held each other tight for minutes without speaking. Only the jerking, halting sobs of the anguished mother could be heard in the room.

When she had a degree of control over her emotions, Anney pulled back from Stephen and locked onto his moist eyes. She studied Stephen's face for a moment, then with resolve said, "Stephen, we have to do something. I don't care what—but something. We can't go on this way."

"What are you suggesting?"

"We have to go up there and get our daughter. Somehow they have to release her from that pit of evil. She is ours, not theirs. She is our daughter . . . and we want her back!"

"Anney, be reasonable. We don't know for sure that she is there." Stephen feared this outburst from Anney. He had lived long enough with this woman of high spirits and determination to know that she was capable of confronting the devil himself with demands and expecting to get results. They left the bedroom.

She walked across the kitchen to the sink, reached for a glass on the shelf, held the glass under the cold running water, filled it, and took a couple of swallows before turning off the stream. She set the glass on the counter, took hold of the counter top with both hands in a firm grip, and spoke firmly, the volume rising to a near shout. "We have to go up to the compound tonight. If we hurry we can be at the gates by early morning. Let's do it, Stephen. I can't sit around here another minute knowing that my daughter is in the clutches of a madman. I can't, Stephen. I just can't!"

Stephen stared at his wife of twenty-plus years. He hadn't expected her to become so completely irrational in her desperation to find Brenda. "What good will it do to go up there? You can't just walk in and look around."

"How do you know we can't? We're her parents. If she is there we have every right to pull her out."

Once again Stephen said, "Be reasonable, honey. This is something for the authorities to handle."

"Reasonable!" Her deep blue eyes were flaming like a natural gas flame kicked up to the highest notch. "What does that mean? I have been reasonable and nothing has worked. I stood by while you and the others went up there and grabbed this Daniel kid. I have stood by all I can. It's time for action. Now."

"You . . . "

Anney waved off Stephen's attempt to explain. "No. Don't give me any explanations. I don't want to hear what we can't do. Give me some answers as to what we can do." She turned from the counter and once again met Stephen's eyes with her own. "Stephen, for heaven's sakes, you are the father. You have to act. Do something to get our daughter back. Do you hear me? Do something!"

Stephen took a deep breath, exhaling slowly and deliberately, then he said, "Honey, do you recall the advice you have given me over the years when I've come home upset, usually with your father?"

"What advice?"

"Breathing. Okay, breathe deep, sweetheart. Breathe in. Breathe out. In. Out. Do it."

"Don't toy with me, Stephen. This is serious, and I'll not have you making light of this life- and-death situation. Do you hear me?" Anney stalked off to the bedroom, fuming within.

"I still say, honey, we don't know that Brenda is even there."

Stephen lay lightly snoring in their king-size bed as Anney shuffled about quietly getting dressed in the dark. She didn't care about make-up. Her blue jeans, a tan blouse and boots would do. She grabbed Stephen's Raiders cap that hung on his side of the walk-in closet. In five minutes she would be ready for the trip. She dreaded going alone on this desperate journey to Jackson Hole, but she felt there was no other way. If she had luck with her, she would arrive at the compound by midmorning, determined to do all she could to gain entrance to that Satan-inspired prison and free her Brenda.

Her plans to take action into her own hands had begun earlier in the evening when Stephen tried to convince her that they needed to sleep on what they should do. They had talked into the night before Stephen finally dropped off to sleep. He had tried all the while to convince Anney to let the authorities handle the problem of freeing Brenda, if in fact she happened to be there. Whatever he and Anney could do would be of no value, and might actually upset the Oracle to the extent that perhaps he would do something harmful to Brenda. Who was to say? Anney was not swayed. She had lain in bed becoming more and more convinced that no one wanted to take matters into his own hands. Sometime during the night she decided to go it alone. She would go up there and take a stand until someone in the compound came out to talk with her, someone who had the authority to release Brenda. She hoped it would be the Oracle himself.

The sun refused to break through the clouds outside the compound. The diffused gray light of mid-morning cast the compound and the surrounding valley in a shadowy, eerie glow. Anney nosed the Jeep Cherokee to within several yards of the main gate and parked squarely in the center of the road. She set the brake and got out. When she slammed shut the door to the car, she looked up at the gate that loomed in front of her. The double steel doors were painted a dull brown which the harsh weather had streaked with a greenish stain. Anney guessed that the gate was at least eight feet high. It struck her how the castles she had visited around Prague had the same forbidding appearance. She was sure that the gate had been constructed to keep people in rather than to keep intruders out.

No one was in sight, though she felt certain that guards were watching her from the side walls of the gate. There was that small, steel door to her left. She decided to pound on it and demand to see Brenda. She stepped up to it and was about to hit her fist on the center of the door, then had a better idea. She looked around, hoping to find something to make her pounding loud and clear. There was absolute silence outside the gate where she now turned to search for some object. She first picked up a dried stick under the alders and pines that lined the left side of the road, then decided to hike up the incline beyond the trees to where there were stones scattered at random across the rise that led to the cliffs beyond. She picked up an oval stone the size of her fist, returned to the steel side door to the compound, and whacked the metal repeatedly.

No one appeared.

She began pounding on the door again. In a demanding voice she shouted, "Open up! I want to talk to someone. Open up! I'm Mrs. Thorn and I want to talk to someone. Open up!"

Anney continued to pound. The sound of the stone hitting metal sent the noise echoing off the cliffs on either side. She kept up her racket for the next ten minutes. With each blow of the rock against the door, she became increasingly frustrated that no one was responding. "Open this thing! Do you hear me?"

This went on. She paused for a few minutes, allowing herself to listen for any response from inside. Nothing ensued. She pounded repeatedly.

It was another ten minutes before the door slid open to expose Reuben, who stared ominously down at her. As the space widened, she suddenly pushed forward, shoving her open hands into Reuben's chest as he gripped the sides of the metal door in an effort to remain on his feet. Her sudden lunge had taken him off guard. She wanted in and he knew it. Behind Reuben one of the young security guards jumped forward and steadied the chief, blocking Anney. He tried to move her back away from the opening. But she grabbed the molding around the door and held her ground.

"I want in. I may have a daughter in here, and if she is, I've come to get her!" she shouted, trying to see over the men and get a look inside the compound. All she saw was another security guard blocking her view. "Do you understand? I want my daughter! And I want her now!"

"Lady, you have no legal right to enter this area," Reuben shouted, inches from Anney's face. "You will have to leave. We know nothing about your daughter. You are trespassing; and if you don't leave, I will be forced to call the sheriff's office and have you arrested." Reuben held firm as Anney continued to shove her way in.

"Good! Call the sheriff. I need his help," she shouted through clenched teeth.

By now, two other security guards had rushed forward. Anney struggled in vain. She was out of breath and red-faced with anger as she found herself again outside the compound and heard the metal door slide shut behind her.

Filled with anger and frustration, Anney snatched up her rock and began pounding again.

No one slid open the gate a second time.

Anney continued to pound for the next ten minutes, then in utter defeat she tossed the rock to the concrete and screamed, "You people will pay for this. I don't give up easily. You'll pay."

There was silence from within.

With no immediate hope, Anney stepped back from the door and surveyed the wall. She moved to the side, hoping to figure out a way to enter. The twelve-foot stone wall extended to the east twenty-five yards where it butted against a sandstone cliff that went vertical two hundred feet. Turning from the base of the cliff, she could see through the leafless trees that the wall stretched out from the main gate to the west perhaps another hundred yards to the high cliffs on the opposite side. Across the top of the far cliffs she could see that someone had constructed what appeared to be a high-wire fence that would prevent anyone from looking down into the compound. She could see that the compound was secure behind walls and that she would not be allowed in.

At the foot of the cliff, she dropped to her knees in total discouragement. "Oh dear God, why?" Tumbling through her thoughts was the question of why, after all that she and Stephen were doing, the Lord had allowed this to happen.

She had come to peace with the Lord in Europe and had found great relief in knowing that she had discovered the gospel of Christ. There had been a certain bliss as she studied the gospel and accepted baptism. She had believed strongly in the power of good and felt that the Lord would sustain her under all conditions. Now she doubted. What kind of twist of fate would open the doors of truth and then slam those doors on Brenda, subjecting the family to grief? Was the Lord testing her?

She glanced up into the grayness of the morning and wondered. All she wanted at this moment was her daughter. Was this too much to ask? "Surely, you being all powerful," she prayed, "can open the door somewhere for me to have my daughter. Don't do this to me. I am pleading for help. Do you hear me? Dear God, what have I done to deserve this horrible situation? Why can't I have Brenda?"

She sat crouched on the cold, sandy incline for a time. Speaking aloud, she approached the Lord from every angle she could possibly imagine. There had to be an answer. There had to be. Suddenly, she looked up to see the main gate open and a larger-than-life Hummer creep through the gate, pause, then with revved-up engine, nudge the front of Anney's Jeep and begin pushing it back from the gate. Though the brake was on and the gears in park, the power of the Hummer was able to send the Jeep back fifteen feet.

Anney stood up and watched for a moment as the Jeep slid backwards. She began running towards the gate that stood wide open. The driver of the military vehicle reversed the gears and sent the Hummer back beyond the main gate inside the compound, and the doors of the gate quickly locked back in place before Anney reached them. They were sealed once again.

She looked back at the Jeep, then up to the top of the gate and began pounding for those inside to open it.

No response.

\* \* \*

"We'll be having the kids for Thanksgiving. I appreciate you taking the time, Samuel, to have this one final session," Bender said, with sincerity.

"Well, we've made some progress. Actually, if I weren't reviewing this with you, I'd be making notes to myself. I have the lecture coming up next week and need the boning up."

"Good. Let's get right into it, then. I'm listening."

"I think we talked about what I call the welcoming in of the Lamanites, didn't we?"

"Some. Let me review, though. You mentioned that the Lamanites will be brought in to the New Jerusalem after the initial construction of the city has taken place. Does that mean they will arrive after the temple has been built in the New Jerusalem?"

"From what I read, it does," Samuel responded. "Of course, I think there will still be plenty to do. It's evident to me that those Lamanites who are worthy will embrace everything presented to them at this wonderful gathering."

"What about the world at that time? What will it be like? I mean, the terrible judgment on the Gentiles will have already taken place."

"Maybe. That is, maybe it will have ended, but I don't know. I do know that the Lord tells us that the House of Israel will be brought in. This means the Lost Tribes will come down to the City of New Jerusalem. Can you imagine the gathering that is going to take place? Oh, to be there."

\* \* \*

It was noon, and the persistent, gloomy clouds still prevailed when Stephen pulled up behind the Jeep. He had surmised where Anney had gone when he awoke at four in the morning. Within minutes he had dressed and had been on his way to Jackson Hole. He drove Anney's aging BMW.

Stephen immediately spotted Anney seated behind the wheel of the Jeep. She had repositioned it in front of the main gate near the same spot as before. This time the front bumper of the Jeep was pressed firmly against the gate. If they opened the gate again, she was prepared to drive forward.

Stephen came up along the driver's side and rapped on the window. Startled, Anney saw Stephen and opened the door. Neither said a word as they looked into each other's eyes. Then Stephen spoke, ''Honey, honey. My dear Anney. Oh, this is such torment for you.''

Anney burst into tears. "Stephen, they won't let me in. I tried, but they won't let me in." She knew it was hopeless for her to enter the compound.

\* \* \*

Stephen sat across from her in the Burger King five miles down the main highway from Jackson.

"I'm so glad I have you away from that gate and safely with me," Stephen responded as he studied Anney's weary features.

Earlier, Stephen had backed the Jeep around from the main Gateway gate and in a giant, determined move nearly dragged Anney to the driver's side and insisted that she follow him away from the compound and head for home. It took another fifteen minutes, as the engine idled, for him to convince her that no one was going to come out of the compound gate and let her in. Anney, with great reluctance, had put the Jeep in drive and followed Stephen to the Burger King in Jackson. He ordered two Whoppers and a malt for himself. Though Anney had not eaten since the night before, the only thing that tempted her was the smell of fresh brewed coffee. She had given it up months ago, but the memory of the effects of caffeine on her body and the aroma that inspired it lingered in her system. How she craved a piping hot cup of black coffee. It was the only thing stirring her taste buds. Her Whopper rested unwrapped on the tiny two-place table top. Stephen wolfed down his burgers and slurped up the strawberry malt, leaving no doubt that he was famished.

Anney had not said a word since Stephen literally insisted she follow him in the BMW.

"I'll drive my own car home." These were the first words Anney had uttered since leaving the walls of the compound.

"Okay," Stephen concurred. He knew she always preferred her car to any other. "Why did you bring the Jeep instead of your Beamer? You never take the Jeep, given a choice."

"Does it matter?"

"Not really. I'm just curious."

"No, what you are curious about is me. Why would I do such a stupid thing as drive up here alone thinking I could somehow find Brenda? That's what you're thinking." She turned her head to look out at the early afternoon bleakness. There were only two other customers in the place.

Stephen observed that the day before Thanksgiving the junk-food business seemed to have a poor showing. People seem to hold off, the better to stuff themselves the next day. He forced his thoughts back to Anney's determination to find Brenda.

"I really thought they would open the gate and let me in to talk to someone, someone who would know whether Brenda was in the compound. I really thought that, Stephen. I did." Anney was speaking more forcefully. This encouraged Stephen. She seemed to be fighting back, the old Anney in charge. "I know you have a hard time understanding my feelings, but I'm her mother. I'm like a lioness with her cub. I will fight to get her back." Anney stared down at her hands, still dirty from the stone she had used to pound the gate. "I felt so all alone. While I was prowling around that fortress from hell, lots of things went through my mind, and one of them was your attitude." Anney lifted her gaze to look deep into Stephen's eyes.

Stephen put down the fragment of his hamburger and placed his left hand over his chest and said, "My attitude? What do you mean?"

"Nothing."

"Yes, something. What do you mean by 'my attitude'? That tone means you think I'm a cop-out. You think I should have been the macho guy you've always thought I was, that I should have rushed up to that compound, torn down the gate like Arnold Schwarzenegger and stormed the Bastille. You think I should have mustered the troops from the sheriff's department, or whoever, and gotten the action going. Right?" Stephen placed both hands on the plastic table top in frustration. "Well, Anney, we have no proof that she is in that compound."

"I didn't say that." Anney wished she had kept her thoughts to herself.

"No, but that's what you meant. You think I'm some kind of wimp. How can you think I don't care about Brenda? What right do you have to accuse me of being a lesser father because I can do nothing at the moment to find Brenda? How can you?"

Tears formed in the corners of Anney's concerned eyes. She knew if she said another word, it would come out wrong. Silence would have to do. Be silent. She still had the presence of thought to realize that Stephen was growing not only impatient with her, but testy in the extreme. She never liked to see Stephen angry, especially at her.

Stephen saw the tears squeeze from Anney's tightly closed eyes and knew he had become too sharp with her. He immediately softened his tone of voice, "I'm sorry, honey. When I got up to go to the bathroom early this morning and you were gone . . . I knew where you had gone. I just knew and I got scared. All the way up here my mind kept pounding away with the thought that if you pushed that crowd out there too far, they would do some wicked thing to you. They are killers."

"Oh, Stephen, oh, Stephen!" Anney pushed the words from her lips with the same torment he had seen in her the day he had told her in San Diego that he had become converted to the LDS Church. It had caused Anney such pain. He knew that the torment Anney felt was like a giant toothache that could not be assuaged. He wished he could retract the word "killers." It was the last thing Anney needed to hear.

"I'm sorry I said that. I don't know what these people are like or whether they would do harm to Brenda. They are a religious cult, and surely some of those inside the compound have a drop of human kindness in their blood. I have to think they have."

Anney used her cheap napkin to wipe her eyes. Silence prevailed while he sat studying her. Finally, he said, "We'd better get back on the road. Are you okay to drive? We can leave the BMW here and have Todd and Max pick it up tomorrow. Why don't we do that? I'll drive you home with me. You need to sleep."

"No. I'm okay. I would never be able to sleep. Not yet. I can drive. The boys won't want to have to come all the way up here." She let the burger rest on the table and stood up. Stephen, still famished, reached across her as she put on her ski jacket and put her Whopper in his coat pocket to scarf down as soon as he was alone in the Jeep.

"You're right. It's not fair to insist they come. Besides, no one knows where we are, and they don't need to." Stephen hoped to avoid telling anyone about the little incident in Jackson Hole.

Anney followed Stephen to the door. "I didn't want to have to go back into the bedroom to get my keys when I left."

"What are you talking about?" Stephen queried as they made their way through the open glass door of the Burger King.

"You asked me why I took the Jeep. The Jeep's keys were on the little rack you mounted on the wall in the kitchen. Mine were not. I didn't want to wake you by rattling my keys on the dresser when I left early this morning."

"Oh, yeah. Okay."

Anney gripped Stephen's arm before he moved away from her in the parking lot to get into his car. "What?"

"Stephen, as long as we're up here, can we go by the sheriff's office? I want to ask him about things."

Stephen felt as if he were on a tight rope. His first mental reaction was to say no. Then he realized how fragile Anney was and relented.

Sheriff Harmon was not in. The deputy at the desk, a man who seemed twice as wide as he was tall, had a cheerful, pink face. Stephen thought he would be able to spot the guy's baby pictures, given the chance. He was uniformed and sat behind an oak desk that fit the scheme of the frontier decor. He was certainly ready to answer all questions except those that counted.

"So when do you expect the sheriff back?" Stephen asked, as he and Anney stood directly in front of the desk.

"All the sheriff said was that he'd be back before the end of the day."

"Well, we can't wait that long," Stephen declared without looking at Anney. He didn't want to spend half the night on the highway to Provo. "Would you please tell him that Mr. and Mrs. Thorn dropped by? We'll be calling him."

"Sure thing."

They left the building and started across the small, paved parking lot to their cars. Just as Stephen neared the rear section of the Cherokee he looked up to see a brown Buick with a red spotlight mounted on the right next to the windshield pulling into a parking spot. From Stephen's side he could read, SHERIFF. Harmon parked in his reserved spot and got out. As he emerged from his car, he noticed the Thorns and in the strong breeze that was sliding off the Tetons he shouted out hello. Behind him came a tall, angular man with a serious expression on his face. It was agent Massey who had stepped out of the passenger side of the sheriff's car.

"Can I help you folks?" Harmon asked with his best folksy, unexpressive smile.

"Sheriff, we are Mr. and Mrs. Thorn. We just thought since we happen to be here in Jackson that . . . well, we'd find out what you know about things out at that compound they call Gateway."

The sheriff listened, then stretched his arm toward Massey and said, "Mr. and Mrs. Thorn, I want you to meet Mr. Massey."

Anney and Stephen extended their hands to the stranger.

"This man is from the FBI in San Francisco." Harmon said. It struck him then that Massey may not have wanted anyone outside of law enforcement in

Jackson to know who he was. Too late. Horn was not the sort who would make a fuss over a slip. Besides, he suspected the Oracle knew that federal law enforcement agents were investigating. He was infamous enough to warrant it.

"We are the parents of a missing girl. We think she may be in Gateway, Mr. Massey."

Massey moved closer to Stephen. He moved his head sideways to eye Anney and said, "Good to see you folks. I just wish I had something positive to tell you about life in the compound. I can understand that you are concerned." He had spent a couple of decades dealing with upset parents and knew well the limits of what he would share with them.

"We want our daughter out of that place. We think she is in there," Anney said, her voice rising alarmingly. Stephen wondered if she was stable enough to meet the two lawmen.

"I can understand, ma'am, but there isn't a whole lot we can do until we have more evidence that something illegal is happening out there. You know all those kids are adults and until we can prove something is going on out of the ordinary, then we have to stay within the bounds of the law. Do you have any proof that your daughter is in there?"

Daniel in New Mexico flashed across Stephen's mind. He wondered if he should reveal all that Burton had told him last night. He didn't want to violate the confidence of Burton, that they would not notify the authorities until they were fairly certain that Daniel was coherent. At least, that had been the agreement.

Anney was not party to what Stephen and Burton had decided about Daniel and his possible evidence as a witness. She looked puzzled, then said, "Stephen, why don't you tell the sheriff about the kid that escaped from Gateway, Daniel? Tell them what he told the doctor was going on in the compound. I think that poor, sick young man needs to tell all he knows to you people."

Harmon's ears seemed to stretch out like tiny satellite dishes primed to receive. "Who is this Daniel?"

Anney opened the discussion. Stephen started to explain about picking up Daniel in Jackson when Massey asked the sheriff if they could step into his office and get a clear picture of what had happened. He was unaware of anyone escaping Gateway.

By the time Stephen and Anney had pulled their cars out of the parking lot at the sheriff's station, Harmon and Massey were on the phone to New Mexico. Massey was not about to wait because some doctor felt that the young man was too disoriented or whatever to reveal what he had witnessed at Gateway.

\* \* \*

Traveling along I-80, trailing Stephen, Anney turned the dials on the Pioneer stereo in her BMW half a mile from the off ramp at Brigham City, headed south. Now that the authorities had something to go on, she felt more confident that she would soon know one way or the other whether Brenda was in Gateway. She was searching for a news station that might give the weather. The clouds were heavy, but no rain or snow had fallen yet. Since leaving Jackson Hole, she had kept the bright red taillights of the Jeep in her vision. Stephen had advised her. He told her they would stop for gas around Brigham City. "If we get separated, there is a Shell station at the off ramp to Brigham City. We'll pull over there and regroup if anything happens. Okay?"

The two-and-half-hour drive to the Brigham City off-ramp gave her time to think about how much Stephen meant to her and that she would not again allow herself to even entertain the thought of Stephen not wanting to get Brenda out of that hell hole. She stopped turning the knob when the announcer on the AM station identified it as KSL News.

"AT THE TOP OF THE HOUR," Anney heard, "WE HAVE A STORY COMING OUT OF TENNESSEE THAT THERE HAS BEEN A MASS SUICIDE IN THE REMOTE TOWN OF BRECKENRIDGE. A GROUP THAT CALLS ITSELF THE 'NEW ORDER FOR GOD' HAS CAREFULLY AND SYSTEMATICALLY COMMITTED SUICIDE OVER THE PAST THREE DAYS. AT LATEST COUNT SIXTY-TWO PEOPLE, MOSTLY MEN, HAVE PARTICIPATED IN A CEREMONIAL SUICIDE. WE WILL HAVE AN UPDATE ON THE SITUATION IN TENNESSEE AS SOON AS WE HAVE MORE INFORMATION."

Stunned, Anney pulled her foot from the accelerator, swerved to the side of the freeway, and stopped the BMW. Stephen, who was about to exit, saw her stop. He hit the brakes. Slowly he reversed the Jeep, looking over his shoulder with his right arm stretched across the bucket seat of the passenger side until he was within five feet of the BMW. As he got out, a three-trailer semi swished by, sending a blast of air that pushed Stephen to the rear of the Jeep. He quickly regained his footing and took several giant strides to the passenger side of the BMW. He opened the door and surveyed the scene. Anney had dropped her head to the steering wheel and was sobbing uncontrollably. He edged into the car and gathered Anney into his arms. He could see that she was verging on a near breakdown. He had never really witnessed a breakdown, but he sensed that anything he might say would add to her stress.

"Anney! Anney, sweetheart," he whispered against her hair. "Are you okay? Answer me. Are you all right?" He suddenly felt weak with relief as her head nodded almost imperceptibly against his lips, signaling that she was okay.

"Why did you stop? Do you feel faint?"

Another nod. She seemed unable to speak. It took minutes before she could tell Stephen what she had heard on the news. He begged her to follow him off the freeway to the Shell station on the east side of the highway where they could leave the Jeep for the boys to pick up the next day. "You are in no shape to drive," he said with a shaky voice. "Do you hear me?"

A half-dozen eighteen-wheelers swished by, rocking the small BMW before Stephen spoke again. "Anney, you have to get hold of your emotions," he pleaded. "Surely God will not allow this to happen to our Brenda. Once again, honey, we don't know exactly where Brenda is."

"You don't know that," she answered at last. "What do we know about that madman back there? How do we know he is not tied in with the group I just heard about in Tennessee? We don't know."

"Hang on, Anney, just hang on. You've been through a lot lately. This whole business about the drugs and all. Somehow you have to hope that things will work out. I have faith that they will."

"Maybe you have, but I haven't." There was a sharpness to her voice that implied that she was not willing to give up her emotional commitment to this possible horrible situation. "I'm sorry, but I happen to be Brenda's mother, and I also happen to think she is in grave danger, wherever she is. Do you know that I have a strong feeling that she is in that compound? That's all I have, but that is enough for me to go crazy looking for her." The voice of the old Anney was surfacing. Her ability to face issues head-on was returning. Stephen heard it and knew it was a good sign that Anney was becoming assertive once again. Good for her. "I'm terribly depressed, and I may be on the edge of some scary happenings in my own mind, but I know one thing: I will see this through, even though my faith in God and the Church is waning. That's the truth, Stephen. It is." Anney removed her forehead from the leather padded steering wheel and looked over at her husband.

"What are you saying?"

She wiped her eyes with the back of her hand and said, "I feel no comfort from the Spirit, or from anything for that matter. God seems so far away. I felt closer to him when I went to my father's services. Why is that?"

"I don't know. I don't have a lot of answers, but I do know that up to the time Brenda went into that compound, we were happier than we ever were before we joined the Church. It doesn't compute in my dizzy head."

Silence filled the car. At last Anney straightened her shoulders, studied the gauges of the idling car, and insisted that she could complete the drive home.

"All right, darling," Stephen said. "I'll follow you. You feel faint or anything, just pull to the side and I'll be right behind you. But first we have to gas up over there. Okay?"

"Yeah. Okay."

Stephen took another look at Anney. She had dark circles under her eyes. His emotions and sensitivity toward her overcame him and he pulled her close again. She responded with a feverish movement, untangling her arms to embrace him. "Anney, it will be over soon, I promise you. I know it will."

# Chapter 17

Stephen had slipped silently out of the master bedroom to avoid waking Anney, who slept in spite of her insistence that she wouldn't be able to when she had crawled into bed after ten last night, shortly after arriving back from her ordeal at the compound. Now Stephen left the house and drove to Samuel's apartment to pick up a disk Samuel had left for him. Samuel had given him a key to the place since he and Stephen spent so much time in the apartment's second bedroom, which Samuel had converted into an office, complete with computer, fax, and phones. It had become a command post for directing things concerning the new Center.

It was after 10:00 in the morning when Stephen returned home from Samuel's. He was expecting Todd and Max anytime. Anney had invited them over for Thanksgiving dinner. Stephen knew it would be a less-than-happy day. Brenda. What about Brenda? The house was silent. Nothing baking, nothing cooking. Where was Anney, he wondered, walking through the kitchen from the garage. Strange.

He peered into the living room, then the family room. Still, no Anney. He opened the front door to look out onto the bare ground that next year would hopefully have a lawn and shrubbery. Still, no Anney. He ran toward their bedroom, feeling a slight concern. He had left her asleep before going to Samuel's for the disk. She never slept beyond 7:00 in the morning, though he knew she had been exhausted the night before. At the top of the stairs he could see through the double doors to the master bedroom that Anney was still in bed. The drapes were drawn, giving a shadowy appearance to the room this midmorning. Stephen thought that Anney must have fallen back to sleep. He quietly walked into the bedroom, not wanting to wake her. But he did want to check on her. When he got to the bedside, he could see that she had her head under the covers, the top of her blond hair barely in view on her pillow.

Though he didn't want to wake her, he felt compelled to reach under the covers and feel her face. As his hand touched her cheek, she scrunched down further in the bed.

"Are you all right, Anney, honey?"

Anney stirred slightly under the covers and spoke in a muffled voice. "No . . . yes . . . I'm not sick . . . but I can't face this day. I can't face that Brenda might be up there in that awful place." The covers remained over her head.

Stephen had bent down to check her, then pulled back. He too was troubled, but not to the extent of remaining in bed, shutting out the world. He shook his head like he hadn't any clue as to why she would retreat this way.

"Honey, you can't let this thing destroy you. We have to keep going."

"I can't, Stephen. I can't. I can't face this day. You'll have to take the boys out for dinner. I can't do it."

He could hear the sobs start. Stephen looked up at the ceiling. He had no idea what to do. Leave her and meet the boys? Stay with her and send the boys away when they arrived? No, he couldn't do that. "Anney, sweetheart, please try. Make every effort possible." Stephen knew that try as he might, he could not embellish the edges to make the situation rosy. It was impossible.

"I don't believe that anymore. Stephen, I'm so scared."

With the word "scared" coming faintly from under the covers, Stephen stepped to the bedside and eased his body close to Anney's, slipping his arms around her shoulders on top of the bed covers. She remained motionless.

\* \* \*

"Why do you think your mom refused to have a blessing last night when your dad asked if we would assist?" Max asked as he removed his sweatshirt and put on a clean rust-red shirt from his semi-orderly closet. He and Todd were nearly ready to go to the Thorns' and decide what to do about Thanksgiving dinner. Stephen had told the fellows last evening not to expect Anney to get excited about the day. Part of the morning the two college students had been studying. They had to keep up their studies, regardless of what was happening with the family. Actually, it was more Todd tutoring Max for an upcoming English exam than Todd doing his own homework. Even though Max was in the bonehead group at UVSC, he was moving to the top of the class with Todd's help. No one ever accused Max of stupidity. Todd always maintained, as he often pumped up his roommate, that it was lack of opportunity that placed him in remedial work. No one could be at the top of his computer class, where Max in fact was, and be a bonehead. It was a game of catch up. This morning had been that kind of session--catch-up.

The subject of Todd's mother had not come up until now. Max wanted to let Todd know that he was behind him in his effort to pull his mother out of the dumps. He felt he needed to know why Todd thought she had refused the proffered blessing the evening before. It had been Todd who asked his mother if he and the others could give her a blessing. Todd and Max had been at the house, concerned that they had not been able to reach Todd's parents. Stephen mentioned nothing to the boys about Anney's flight to Wyoming in the middle of the night. Stephen simply said they had been out.

"You want me to pitch you a theory on why I think my mother is acting the way she is?"

"Todd, you don't have to pitch me anything. And I know it's none of my business, so I'll butt out."

Todd was in shorts, leaning against the edge of his desk. He was ready to pull on his jeans. "Max, my mom's psyche in this thing with Brenda is stretched to the very limits. I don't know how much more she can take. But I do know that if she doesn't feel like having my dad and me give her a blessing, that is her business."

"But Todd, . . . nothing."

"What?" Todd let go of the desk and moved around so he could see Max's face. "What were you going to say?"

"I said I would butt out and I mean it."

"No. I don't want you to clam up in this thing. I need to know what you would do if you were me, or what you think my mother should do."

"Okay, but don't take me wrong. You want my opinion? I'll give it to you." Max studied Todd's features a moment. "If it were my mother and I really wanted her to get over this, then I would go over there and sit down with her and tell her straight out that I wasn't leaving until she got a blessing. That's what I would do." Max moved his head from side to side. "Your mom's a great lady. I got to know her a little bit on the ship. She is a sensitive woman with brains. I think—and it's just my wild thought—but I think she will listen to you, Todd. You are her prize kid. She puts a lot of stock in what you say."

"Thanks, but she puts more stock in what my dad says, and he can't get her to listen. No. I'm afraid you don't know my mother."

"Do you?"

"What kind of dumb question is that?"

"Okay, okay. I said what I was thinking, and you don't want to hear from me anymore, so . . . "

"You're right, Max. I'm going to see my mom and get her to have us bless her."

"All right, man. Go for it!" Max shouted. "But not me. I'll stay out of it. You just drop me off somewhere along the way—the juice bar or someplace that's open on Thanksgiving—then pick me up on your way back."

A knock came on their bedroom door. The door opened a crack. "Mom, Dad, can I come in?"

"Sure, Todd. Come in."

At the sudden appearance of Todd, Anney pushed the sheet off her head and raised up on her elbows. Todd came around to her side of the bed and sat down next to her. "Hi, Mom." He reached down and kissed her cheek. "I missed you not being in the kitchen. I'm still your little boy who loves your apple pie."

Anney's face contorted. She reached up and pulled Todd to her breast and sobbed, "Oh, Todd, what have I done? Of course you're my boy. You are so dear to my heart. What have I done to you? I've lost Brenda, but I have to keep you. What have I done?"

Steven scooted across the bed and encircled both of them with his arms. The three held each other for several minutes, tears rolling down all their cheeks. It was sometime later, after a long discussion, that Todd asked Anney if he and Stephen could give her a blessing.

Todd felt that if he was to convince his mother to have a blessing, he needed to express it in his own get-to-the-point fashion. "You know, Mom, that I'm an elder, just like Dad. We have to rely on each other."

"Yes, honey, I know." Anney could sense what her precious young man she loved so much was leading up to. Should she disappoint him a second time and refuse to have a blessing?

"Mom. Can we give you a blessing?"

The very tone that Todd used, the innocence of his demeanor, the little boy that was coming out melted her heart. She could not sit there and refuse her own son. Through her tears, Anney nodded her consent.

"Okay, I'm not sure I have this down, but let's do it," Todd said, pouring a good amount of oil on his mother's head as she sat in the winged chair in the living room. Stephen stood behind him.

"Don't worry, son. The Lord will understand. I will help you."

"I remember seeing this done. Well, we all did on the ship, but I saw another blessing of health a couple of weeks ago. I was asked by this girl who was sick to stand in with the Elder's Quorum presidency. But I've never done it on my own."

"Place your hands on her head, and I'll help you with the words if you don't remember," Stephen assured Todd with great pride in his son.

"Like this?" Todd asked, not at all sure of the proper approach to something so sacred.

"Right. Good. Now, you're anointing, which means you want to use this holy oil for the anointing of the sick in the household of faith. The bishop said that, above all, do it by the power of the Holy Melchizedek Priesthood and close the anointing in the name of Jesus Christ."

"How do you know so much? You've never done it, either."

"I know, but I'm your father and I'm supposed to know. No, the bishop took me through this three times on the phone this morning."

By now Anney was smiling at her two men fumbling about with the clumsiness of boys trying to work out a math problem.

Todd completed the anointing and quickly stood back to let his father move in.

"Now, you put your hands on top of mine or on part of your mother's head." Todd placed his hands atop Stephen's and Stephen sealed the anointing with his own special wording. He repeated his priesthood authority twice. Partway through the blessing, Stephen suddenly felt that the hand of the Lord was silently guiding him in this sublime moment. The words came slowly but firmly from Stephen's lips. He no longer felt that he was doing something for the first time. It was as if he had done this before. He knew he hadn't, at least not in this life. In the blessing he assured Anney that she would have the strength to make it through this trying time. He also broke into a prayer and asked his Heavenly Father to watch over the whole family and to especially comfort Brenda. Words seemed to fail Stephen at this point in the blessing. He paused and pondered while the other two waited for him to continue. In a loud voice that startled Todd, Stephen uttered, "And we bless you, honey, that the influence of the Evil One will leave your mind and body."

Todd raised his head to study his father. Had his father actually commanded some evil being to come out of his mom? Was she, in fact, possessed? He had heard about such blessings pronounced upon individuals, but he had never thought he would be part of the action that would drive out an evil influence. Todd accepted the reality of the situation and lowered his head in agreement. If Satan had part in this, then it was right that his dad rid his mom of that influence.

He pronounced the blessing upon her head in the name of Jesus Christ, then ended it with an amen.

Todd lifted his hands off Stephen's. Stephen left his hands in place on Anney's crown. For more than a minute he stood there, pondering what he had said. A spiritual charge had coursed through his entire body. He was reluctant to let it pass so quickly. He wanted to relish it and to cherish the feeling. He had never in his life experienced anything so spiritual, nothing quite like this moment. He thought to himself that if this is the joy of the gospel, there is little else in life to compare with it. It was the Spirit. Yes, the Spirit of the Lord was in the room. Most definitely.

Anney had dropped her head and her blond hair swept forward; the hands went to the eyes to hold back the flood of tears that were streaming down her face. She couldn't speak. Stephen had released her from something she knew was evil. Of course . . . she believed in Christ.

A tenuous thread of thought linked her back to what she had endured these past several days. Then the evil she had felt entirely faded. Anney let her mind break free of the dreary restraints of her tired flesh. Her mind began to soar, receiving insights into a more glorious future. She explored for a moment comforting thoughts she felt were beyond her ability to comprehend. No more teetering thoughts. All seemed clear now. This new spirit of hope that came over her appeared more textured and intense than the evening in the mountains of Eastern Europe when she had listened to the Spirit bear testimony to her soul. Her thoughts for the moment seemed so brilliantly integrated. She felt enraptured. Something had left her.

Yes, things would work out. Generous portions of hope surged through her thoughts as she wept. She felt Stephen move his head down on top of her crown where the olive oil glistened. They remained tightly embraced for so long, Todd wondered if his mother was relieved or burdened by what he and his father had performed.

Todd could see she was thrilled when Anney finally lifted her face and reached her left hand out for Todd to embrace her as well. Anney was still not up to fixing a meal. Stephen quickly told Todd that they would find a place open and bring back something. "Boston Market is open today. Let's go get some of their takeout. . . . Oh, by the way, where's Max?" Todd explained that he had dropped him off at the mall.

\* \* \*

"Stephen, hurry. You know that FBI agent we met yesterday, Massey? He's on the phone and wants to talk to you." Stephen slammed shut the Jeep's door and rushed into the kitchen as Anney held open the door. Todd and Max followed with the styrofoam boxes of turkey, stuffing, mashed potatoes, gravy--the works.

"He wants a clear picture of Brenda. He said to fax it to him and to that doctor in New Mexico. I already have her senior picture, the one on the piano. I'll take it out of the glass. Hurry. Tell him we can fax it right away."

"He must know something. Good!" Stephen cried, as he lifted the kitchen phone off its wall cradle and nearly shouted. "Yes, Mr. Massey. This is Stephen Thorn. What's happened?"

\* \* \*

Samuel and Katherine arrived at Boise's air terminal by one in the afternoon, about the same time Stephen was transmitting the fax to Massey and Mucranski from his home office.

Samuel's sons and grandchildren were all there to greet them as they came walking briskly through the gate from their commuter flight, a flight that had taken less than an hour. Getting last-minute seats on the Southwest flight was nothing. By noon on Thanksgiving Day, most people had already arrived at their destinations.

Hugs and kisses were bestowed upon Samuel, who played the role of grandfather to the hilt. Katherine could tell he loved it. His romantic little granddaughters were fascinated with Katherine. They had heard their grandfather talk about the lady who lived in a penthouse in San Francisco, the one who had invited him for a vacation on a yacht in the South Pacific. They had not listened to the part about the group researching and discussing the whereabouts of the surviving Nephite nation. Katherine appeared to them as regal and as beautiful as Samuel had described her on his last visit home, when the entire family had gathered to welcome their world-traveling grandfather back to Boise. Now he was home for the holiday, and this time he brought this stunning lady who wore a fur coat—her beaver jacket—with its soft, light tones.

One of the younger granddaughters, Madison, whom Katherine suspected was five, tugged on the beaver and said, "Are you going to marry Grandpa?"

Katherine looked up at the rest, who had happened to overhear Madison's innocent question, and answered with a little laugh, "Well, little ones get right to the point, don't they?" Samuel's face turned red, but he smiled. It pleased him that there was no feigned denial in Katherine's response. Soon the whole gang swept through the relatively small terminal to the curb where two vans waited to carry them all back to Samuel's stately home off the ninth hole in the exclusive, gated community the developers had named The Plantation.

Katherine loved the setting of Samuel's large, country French home that sat fifty yards back from the Boise River. It was surrounded by trees that had been growing for the past half century and more. When the builders had cleared the lot to lay the foundation, they had left the marvelous old cottonwood trees untouched. Now, of course, the leaves were gone, but the atmosphere of country living within the city limits of Boise permeated the entire neighborhood of upscale homes. Little Madison tagged along as Samuel took Katherine to the river's edge and strolled with her and the kids along the banks to the ninth hole and back to the house. The storm that hit Jackson Hole earlier had skirted Boise, and the fall sunshine spread its glory across the yellow-green lawn and streamed through the floor-to-ceiling windows off the kitchen-family room.

"Your wife must have enjoyed this beautiful spot," Katherine said as they neared the back terrace where covered lawn furniture stood next to bare planter boxes, waiting peacefully for summer to reappear.

The mention of "wife" and not "Margaret," a name Samuel was certain Katherine remembered, was not lost on him. He knew that Katherine was trying to picture his wife here in her proper place. For his part, at long last he was ready to put the past on the shelf of life, to be recalled on very special occasions, but not to intrude on the very real present.

"Mommy said not to interrupt you and grandpa while you were talking," said a darling, dark-haired little girl of perhaps six.

"Oh, honey, you're not interrupting us," Katherine said. "Go ahead. What did you want to say?"

"Well . . . if you marry Grandpa, will he live at your house or at this house? I want him to live here. . . . And you, too. Is that okay?"

Katherine knelt down on one knee next to the beautiful child. The concrete felt cold to her skin. A stiff breeze blew across the terrace, skittering leaves along the brick wall that led to the expansive lawn. She answered clearly and with sensitivity for the child's feelings. "You know . . . oh . . . let me see, you are . . . "

"Karen. I'm Karen. Don't you remember? I told you my name in the car."

"Yes, yes. You are Karen. You know, Karen, you remind me of Belle in *Beauty and the Beast*. Did you see that wonderful movie?"

"Yes," Karen replied, her eyes shining. "I got the video for my birthday last year. Do you really think I look like Belle? I like you. What do I call you? I forgot your name, too."

Samuel looked down, noticing how carefully Katherine had sidestepped the question about where they would live if they married.

"You can call me Katherine. Sometimes, when I was a little girl like you, my friends called me Kathy."

"Oh, I like Kathy. I have a friend named Kathy in my Primary class. I'll call you Kathy."

Katherine stood up and met Samuel's eyes. She read them clearly. *I love you*, they said. Her response was mutual.

Samuel had two sons who ran the lumber business, but there was no work talk at the dining table. The girls had served the feast buffet style. The table was too crowded with plates, silverware, stemmed glasses, and a centerpiece to make room for food. Everyone had filled their plates from the buffet table before sitting down to eat. As head of the family, Samuel had offered grace before everyone began eating. There were twenty-two present, and that didn't include Samuel's other children who were having Thanksgiving dinner with in-laws. Samuel sat at the head of the table and Katherine sat on his right. When the house was new, he had ordered the specially crafted table to accommodate twenty people when all the leaves were inserted. The tablecloth had also been a special order from a linen shop in Salt Lake City over two years before, just a few months before Samuel's wife died of cancer.

With her keen sense of perception, Katherine noticed a reserved attitude among the adults around the long dining table. They were certainly cordial . . . but perhaps wary would best describe their demeanor. In fact, from the moment Katherine shook hands with Samuel's sons at the airport and later met the daughters and daughters-in-law in the kitchen, she had sensed that she had been judged unfit material for the Meyers clan.

Samuel's oldest son, a bishop and president of the family lumber business, attempted to put Katherine at ease, but fell short of the mark. Perhaps it was the reserved way he spoke or the pointed questions he asked about her life and how she had met his father that sent signals of concern along the table. "Katherine, we understand that your former husband was a popular televangelist. Just what is a televangelist?"

The question had a bit of a barb to it. No one needed to tell her that their father was a card-carrying, dyed-in-the-wool Mormon of the first water. She knew as much, and, up to this moment, it hadn't really been an issue. Oh sure, she wondered at times if she could ever accept the strict moral codes that Samuel lived to the letter. However strict, they were part of what had endeared him to her. Maybe she was mellowing in her advancing years. Whatever, his straight-laced morals had never seemed to interfere with their affection for one another. She felt suddenly that Samuel was far more eclectic in his views of mankind than this enthroned son who seemed to be guarding the reputation of the family's Mormon heritage.

None of his children had directly referred to the relationship that had developed between Katherine and Samuel. Perhaps nothing would be said—at least on this visit—about such a religiously unmatched duo, but she could see that sooner or later it would come into play.

* * *

Thanksgiving Day in the cave at Gateway meant nothing. It crossed Martha's mind that it was the day of the traditional holiday only because Jeremiah was watching one of the football games traditionally played on this day. She had no interest in football or any other televised sport. She left the communications center shortly after taking a seat where she had hoped to have a casual conversation with Jeremiah. He was too wrapped up watching the pounding flesh on the screen to talk.

Martha had looked in on Brenda to check her progress. It was the four-hour sleep period for the young inmate. Martha would roust her in another half-hour and pretend anger. It was not always easy for Martha to act out the parts she had scripted for her programming of youth.

Perhaps it was the wall of the cave when she stepped out of the prefabricated building into the vast cavern that struck her as a bleak way of life. She had been raised with the tradition of Thanksgiving. Granted, her father, a widower, never provided a fancy meal on this day, but in his own way he celebrated the day. They usually ended up in a fast-food outlet and had hamburgers or some other variety of junk food in tribute to the day of feasting. She remembered that the last time she sat across from her father she had been fourteen. He died that year, and she had ended up with an aunt in the Bronx. Some life. Two years later she was on the streets and tied in with a group of flower children who took her with them to San Francisco. It was the end of the flowering era, but the beginning of life with Dr. Von Heinrik, whom she met in Union Square at a protest rally. He took her off to Central America and later to South America. What a life. It seemed to her now that she never had been a kid.

What if she had been raised like Brenda? Would she be a mother now? Where would she be? Perhaps she would have a comfortable home somewhere in the suburbs, a couple of children, a decent husband, and above all . . . a life. How much longer could she go on with this insane people-programming? How long?

Her thoughts were interrupted when she saw the Oracle stepping briskly through the cave, bound for the communications room. He noticed Martha next to the interior building and waved. It was not so much a "hello" as a "come on in with me" type of signal with his hand. Martha knew the signal well. It was the Oracle's way of directing her to join him and others in a conference session. She pulled herself away from the wall and followed him inside the center.

"So, none of you knew this guy in Tennessee?" the Oracle asked after getting comments from Jeremiah, Martha, and Reuben who joined them after five minutes of discussion. "It was a stupid thing to do. Look at the thriving organization he had. All those dedicated people, and he up and leads them in song and death. I heard about that old man while I was still living in Delaware. As a matter of fact, I think I was on a panel with him, but I can't remember. No, I know I was. It was one of those discussions about religious groups, and Larry King had us on his show. Yeah, he was there. I thought then he was a little weird." The Oracle was swinging his head back and forth in bewilderment about the madman in Tennessee who had led his people in mass suicide.

The Oracle looked up to meet Martha's eyes. She wanted to be anywhere but in this room with this man she utterly detested. "Martha, you toy with people's minds. Tell me. How was this leader able to convince his people that they could escape to a better life and get them to go along with him?"

Martha didn't hesitate in her answer, "Loyalty to the man. It happened in South America with the Jones people. He must have held them under his spell for years. And when he told them it was time to move to a new, higher level of life somewhere out there," she pointed up, "they followed him to their deaths."

"You may be right. But it wasn't the way to do it. From what I hear on the news, it was some sort of poison. That is no way to go. Armageddon, fiery destruction—that is the way to go. Myself, I believe God will come down and visit us personally. Whatever he asks of me and mine, that we will do."

* * *

Stephen checked on Anney three times during the day. Though she'd had the blessing she was exhausted and Stephen knew she needed the rest. He tried to watch the Cowboys game on TV with Todd and Max who stretched out on the newly laid carpet in the family room. He finally left the family room to the boys and their game and decided to review the project's financial figures that he had picked up at Samuel's earlier. As he crossed the living room, he heard the phone ring in the kitchen. He quickly raced for it to prevent it from disturbing Anney.

It was Samuel calling from Boise. "I didn't get a chance to talk to you yesterday. I called around and only got the machine," Samuel said in his upbeat voice. "I thought you might want to know the number here at my place in Boise so you can reach me this weekend if anything pops."

"It's good of you to call, Samuel, but I think I have your number in my study. Did Katherine go with you to your place? I tried to call her this morning and got no answer."

"Yeah, we're having a great time. My family seems to like her."

"Why wouldn't they?"

"Well, for a starter she's not a member of the Church, and they think we are practically married."

Stephen knew that Samuel was referring to a long family tradition of temple marriages. It would never set well with Samuel's clan to marry outside the temple. To Stephen it made little sense that the location of their marriage would have any bearing on their romance. Besides, Stephen felt certain that Katherine would soon join the Church and that would fix the problem. Oh well. "I understand what you're saying. Just reinforce the fact that Katherine is a quality person."

\* \* \*

It was late afternoon when Katherine slipped up to the guest room where she was to spend the night. Great quantities of food had been consumed, the dishes were washed, and some of the families had already left for their own homes. She breathed a sigh of relief that the rest of them would soon be gone, that is, all except three of the grandchildren who would be sleeping over for the fun of it. It wouldn't have been proper for Katherine and Samuel to spend the remainder of the weekend alone together in the large house. It wouldn't have bothered Katherine, but she understood that it was not acceptable for Samuel.

A faint tap on the solid-core paneled door interrupted Katherine's thoughts. "Come in. Please come in," she called.

Through the door came one of the grandsons, awkward, thin. Katherine recalled that his name was Mark. Because of his narrow face, buckteeth, protruding ears and wide grin, Katherine remembered him best of all the grandsons around the table. She guessed he was not much older than nine, if that. "Well, Mark, I thought you were never going to speak to me," Katherine said, smiling. "Would you like to come in and visit?"

"Do you know how to play Uno?"

"Of course. Do you have a deck of cards?"

"In the playroom in the basement. Want to come play with us?"

"Sure I do. What fun!"

The children seemed to like her and giggled all the way through the first game. Katherine told them how she used to play Uno with mentally challenged children at St. Mary's Health Center in San Francisco, where she was a volunteer. "Some of those kids are as good at winning as you." Katherine was careful not to win. She knew enough about children to know that they reveled in winning. Halfway through the third game, Mark's mother shouted from the top of the stairs for him to come. The family was ready to leave. It crossed Katherine's mind to go up with Mark and say goodbye to that small family: the bishop, and his wife, and two children. She soon had second thoughts.

"I'm coming," Mark shouted, looking across the card table at Katherine. "I wish I didn't have to go. Are you going to be here tomorrow? Maybe Mom will bring me back over tomorrow."

"Maybe not, too," said Mark's cousin Dick, then ducked his head. He was about eight or nine as well. Dick had just come downstairs to join the Uno players. "I just heard your mom say that she wasn't coming back to this house as long as *she* . . ." Dick's face suddenly turned red and he stopped in mid-sentence. Katherine peered closely at the embarrassed boy, the unspoken words clamoring in her mind.

"You be quiet, Dick," said Mark in a threatening tone. "A lot you know."

Katherine stood up with dignity and walked Mark to the bottom of the stairs where she said goodbye and touched his shoulder. "Thank you, Mark, for sticking up for me, but I think perhaps I'm not as welcome here as I had hoped."

"I like you, Katherine. Sorry he hurt your feelings."

Katherine turned away. She didn't want Mark to see the tears gathering in the corners of her eyes. Angry at herself, she blinked them away. *Why in the world had she consented to come? Thanksgiving was a family time, and she had been an intruder. But would there ever have been a good time to meet Samuel's family?* Katherine was certain there would not.

As soon as she heard the door close behind the last of the families, Katherine hurried upstairs for her things. Good thing she hadn't had time to unpack yet. It would hurt Samuel, but she could not stay the night in this environment. It wasn't working. It never would.

When Katherine walked down the stairs with suitcase and makeup case in hand, she dreaded confronting Samuel. Using the phone in the guest room, she had already called a taxi as well as the airline to make reservations on a plane from Boise to Seattle and a connecting flight that would get her to San Francisco by midnight—home, where she belonged. She waited on the line for confirmation, but they couldn't give her one due to heavy booking. She was chagrined by her foolish actions—buying the townhouse in Provo, and pushing her way into others' lives. Well, she had learned her lesson. As hard as it would be to reject Samuel's pleas, Katherine resolved to remain firm in her decision to go home. Now!

She was a lonely figure stepping to the tarmac from the airport van that stopped at the wingtip of the prop plane . Katherine had generously made the arrangements from the counter of Boise's air terminal when she arrived from Samuel's. She wanted to travel solo, no one to see her red eyes, her broken heart. Besides, the one flight to Portland that would connect her with a flight to San Francisco was overbooked. People were eager to get back home after the holiday feast. The charter service had assured her that a prop plane was available within an hour. They also reminded her that this was considered an express service that required an additional fee. The fee was the least of her concerns.

Misty, cold, and nearly void of people, the noncommercial area of Boise Airport seemed to be perched on bleak rock suspended in space. Visibility was okay for takeoffs and landings, but barely. When Katherine had arranged for the last-minute charter at the VIP counter, she knew she was fortunate to find a plane and pilot on a day when usually there was little need for a charter. The pilot who spoke to her on the telephone assured her that he had the fastest prop plane available, and that he could whisk her to Oakland in less than an hour and a half. Fine.

The airport attendant stuffed Katherine's red-leather weekend case inside the left storage compartment, then stood back to take Katherine's hand as she graciously climbed the eight steps up to the cabin and disappeared inside. It was a nine-seater in the passenger section. The scent of new leather, stained steel gray, invaded her senses. She chose the seat second from the rear on the left. As she moved to the rear, the pilot—blond, fortyish, thin, with a serious face— leaned to his right and turned his head to see Katherine seat herself and buckle up. He shouted through the opening between the cockpit and cabin, "Ma'am, I'm Cary O'Tool. I'll be your pilot on this flight. Thank you for the opportunity to escort you to the Bay Area. If you wish a drink, there is a small refrigerator cabinet behind you in the rear. Help yourself." He studied her face for a moment when she smiled a cool acknowledgment. He sensed that his passenger was not interested in unnecessary conversation. Katherine was certainly not in her form. He resumed his position and asked the tower for clearance to approach Runway B for takeoff.

Once in the air, the twin prop leveled off at 30,000 feet—above the clouds. Behind the aircraft a purple curtain of clouds spread to the eastern horizon; in front the orange afterglow of sunset illuminated the silver craft. Katherine stared out the small oval window, looking at nothing. Bleak-hearted, she realized that she had acquired a new definition of personal fear—denying love, denying the most longed-for, precious person in her universe. She had walked away from something so dear to her heart, so elusive in her life, that she now trembled inside at the thought.

She tilted her head back and breathed hoarsely. This new-found fear caused her to be terribly dry. She released the belt, slid out of her seat, and moved wearily to the cabinet that stood snug along the cabin wall at the rear. Inside the small refrigerator, on the top rack, she saw a small plastic bottle of Evian. She retrieved it, retook her seat, and buckled the belt once again.

Sipping the pure spring water did not douse the burning void in the pit of her stomach. It couldn't. The pain burned. It stabbed. It gnawed. There was no relief for her brand of pain—none at all. She had never in her life been jerked up so sharply by her sense of doing right for the right reasons. It was right to not deceive one she loved. It was right to turn her back on pursuing a phony life with one she loved. She would have to live with her decision to choose the right. Additionally, she had never experienced quite the personal chagrin she had endured earlier in the afternoon. And yet, the hurt Samuel's family had inflicted on her was really nothing compared to the hurt she now felt at leaving Samuel. Her mind whirled with regret. She had somehow managed to walk away from the single, most-desired person in her life. But it wasn't a point of pride to her—not now, not yet, not with these feelings that plunged her to the bottom rung of hope. She couldn't remember ever being so heartsick as she felt right this very moment. She had felt on the verge of nausea since leaving Samuel's front doorstep. Now, even breathing was an effort. She sat thinking, groping along the lining of her brain, bewildered that she was able to make the decision to leave. Granted, Samuel's children helped her make that move. She wanted to prevent the pain but saw no proper way to do so. What would ease her mind while dredging up the day's disaster? This pain in her heart seemed to have a will of its own. She could not bring herself to indulge in some drugged escape by drinking. It would not be right. If Samuel had done nothing else, he had given her a sense of doing the right thing. She would honor her desire to be more like him, though he would not be there to offer any further instruction on just how to do that. Samuel had not distanced himself from her; rather, she was now distancing herself from him in an effort to do what she sincerely felt was right. So noble. . . . So stupid.

Disturbingly, her fingers, gripping the plastic water bottle, trembled. She squeezed the sides until they caved in and water spilled from its mouth. Would she ever get through this stage of emotional agony? The thoughts that now erupted troubled her as much as the loss of Samuel. If the plane crashed. . . . If only—of course, except for the pilot, who in some miraculous way would escape injury, leaving her behind—then she would welcome a crash that would take her life. What a horrible thought. Yet, it was her thought. And though she was ashamed to admit it aloud, she thought it nevertheless.

* * *

Samuel let the phone ring until the answering machine picked it up. It was Burton checking in from New Mexico. "Call me, Sam. I have some interesting news to share with you. We have the goods on our boy in Gateway; I hope to shout we do. I'm at . . ." Sam could hear Thom read off the phone number of the Days Inn where he was sleeping for the night.

Samuel listened to the message again and decided to wait a few more minutes before following up on the call. All Samuel could think about was Katherine. Watching her get into the back seat of that taxi had nearly ripped his heart out. She had hardly said a word when she told him she was going home to San Francisco. What she did say had seared his heart. She had tipped her lovely head to the side and whispered, tears slipping down her cheeks, "It isn't going to work, Sam. I come from a different world than yours. I'm not a Mormon. Your daughter-in-law is right. This woman does not belong in the Meyers household. Goodbye, Sam. I love you."

Samuel had stood immobile while the cab driver closed the door and Katherine nodded that she was ready. What had his daughter-in-law said? Why, all of a sudden, did Katherine seem as cold as the Boise River out back? What on earth had happened? He had already been dazed when Katherine walked quietly downstairs and made her unexpected exit. His mind was reeling from an intense discussion with his son, which had taken place while Katherine played Uno with the children.

"Dad, *Dad!"* Robert had begun. "What are you doing? How can you possibly think of marrying a nonmember?" When Samuel had extolled Katherine's virtues and flatly stated that he loved her, Robert had sat still for a long time. Finally, he had said, "Don't you remember how upset you and Mom were when Barbara wanted to marry Rafe Willard? He was a great kid. He came from a wonderful family. He was sharp, had a full scholarship to Northwestern Dental School. By the world's standards, he was a terrific catch for her . . . and she loved him. Don't you remember what you said to her? . . . And what message will you be sending to your grandchildren? Think about it, Dad."

He was suddenly plunged back a dozen years. And, yes, he could remember what he had said to Barbara. He might as well have been watching a video of the scene. He had taken her icy hands in his and looked with love and anguish into her ashen face. "Oh, Barbara, sweetheart," he had pleaded, "I wonder if you can even imagine how totally you are woven within the fabric of the Church. Right now you are caught up in the excitement of romance with this young man. But life has a way of settling down to plain, day-to-day effort. Problems will arise. Rafe will sometimes want you to do other things on the Sabbath, and you will drift away. You don't think so now, but it happens.

"And what will you do when your children are ill? Won't it break your heart if their father cannot lay his hands upon their downy little heads and give them a blessing? It will hurt you when your younger sister marries in the temple and you can't be inside with the rest of the family. You will feel shut out, not just from the temple, but in a sense from the family. Just think of it. *Whenever* there is a marriage—a niece or nephew—you will not be able to be with the family in that most sacred place. My child, you think that there will never be another love for you, but you are wrong. You are so young and beautiful. A fine young priesthood holder will surely come along. He will love you, and he will believe all that you believe. I beg you, *please* have faith and wait for that day."

Samuel sat in the darkness of the living room. His grandchildren who had stayed to spend the night were engrossed in a movie in the family room. They were oblivious to his deep sorrow; Samuel was grateful for that. He wanted no one to see him in such despair. Hell must be something like this, he thought—great longing that consumes and no possible way to find relief.

He stared at the streetlights that were aglow out the large bay window as he recalled Katherine's words over and over again in his mind. She was right, of course. They were on two separate tracks in life. If she never understood the importance of the gospel of Jesus Christ, what kind of relationship could they hope to have? Purely a worldly thing. She would have to embrace the gospel to truly understand his deepest feelings and become a part of his soul. If he allowed himself to marry her for time only, without her commitment to the gospel, it would pull down the moral fiber of his very being. "She's right," Samuel whispered to himself. "I've been kidding myself. She does come from a different world."

He thought again of Barbara. She had been an obedient daughter. She had followed his counsel and broken off with Rafe. Just as he had promised, another fine young man had come along, and she had married him in the temple with all the family gathered around. They had four darling children now. She seemed happy enough . . . didn't she? She didn't have that old sparkle in her eyes, but that was because she was older . . . wasn't it? Who would have believed that Rafe would get involved with Mormon students in Chicago and join the Church? He even filled a mission. Samuel's heart grew heavier and heavier. He understood Barbara's feelings better now.

In the depths of his remorse, Samuel's heart finally got the upper hand. *Go after her. At least confront the issue. Make every effort possible to change whatever is dividing you.* Yes, he would fly to San Francisco first thing in the morning. The grandchildren would have to cut their weekend short. He would call their parents and explain that he had to see Katherine. They would have to handle that information the best way they could.

He knew he would not sleep well tonight. But, regardless, tomorrow he would knock on Katherine's door. And when it opened, he would shove his foot in it. He thought he ought to wear a stout shoe that could take the abuse. He suddenly felt that, like the shoe he would wear, he could take a little abuse too, if the reward was good enough. The reward would be good enough, all right. It was Katherine.

.

Feeling better, Samuel arose from the sofa and walked across the hall to his study. He was ready to return Burton's call. He was, in fact, ready to take on the world. He would go to Katherine and get her to see that she was a special spirit of Heavenly Father—a very special daughter of God.

* * *

"When will you be back in Provo? Saturday?" Burton wanted to know as he spoke with Samuel by phone.

"Sorry, Thom, but I have to fly out to San Francisco and see Katherine."

"Isn't she there with you? I thought the two of you were going to spend Thanksgiving together."

"We did spend part of the day together; then something personal happened and she took off. I'm going to follow her in the morning and hopefully put things back together." Samuel wondered why he was telling Burton about his personal foibles. He hardly knew the man.

"I can only tell you one thing, Sam, and I tell you this from experience: Women are very difficult to understand. They are not constructed the same way as men. I say no more. Anyway, will you call me sometime tomorrow from San Francisco? Please, Sam, I need support."

"Okay, I'll call. But I may stay in San Francisco for a few days. For heaven's sake, call the authorities, Thom. At least include that in your plans. Of course. They have your number as well as Stephen's." Samuel paused, then said in a near whisper, as if there were ears in the room, "You know, Thom, we've got to get to the bottom of this, and not merely to satisfy ourselves that the person responsible is put away. We're dealing with a deranged person. Those guys in the compound could find out that it was us who picked up Daniel. We really don't know whether we were seen at the shopping mall that night. If they think we are investigating this thing full bore, our lives could be in danger."

"I've thought of that, too, Samuel. You're right; we've got to move."

"I'll say, and move fast. Is there anything else I can do to help." Burton wanted to mention a couple of other points, though held back and said he'd be in touch.

# Chapter 18

Wasting no time, Thom Burton had either been on the phone or pounding away on his computer's keyboard seeking more information on the Grand Oracle and trying to reach college officials to find out more about Daniel as a student. He knew the FBI was moving faster, but he refused to wait for their investigation. He wanted to make certain he had the facts as well. He had researched from his office in downtown Salt Lake City late into the night. Since Dr. Mucranski put him on to a new angle that revealed more about the Oracle, Thom wanted to know everything that had been written up on this self-styled prophet. This evening he was able to contact two of his favorite journalist friends: Morris in Oakland and Shaver in Los Angeles, plus a Seattle TV reporter that Morris had suggested. All had done background research on the Oracle, but had not run a story. Morris had told him about their work earlier. They gladly shared the information they had uncovered about the activities of the Oracle over the last thirty years. Before that time the Oracle had lived a secluded life on his family's estate in Maryland, and there was little, if anything, out of the ordinary in his life. After that, however, the trail of cult involvement spread from South America to the Orient and back to Wyoming. Burton began to spot a pattern of behavior on the part of the Grand Oracle in his involvement with the cult movement worldwide.

Thom surmised by late evening that the leader at Gateway had sought out other cult leaders who seemed to predict some future happening, the Doomsday boys. Though not finished with his research, he shut down his computer by 11:00 in the evening. It had been a long day. He reasoned that since tomorrow, the day after Thanksgiving, was considered a semi-holiday, he would have time to continue his research in the morning. Little else was happening in the world of news this long weekend. He had decided that first thing in the morning he would contact Stephen Thorn and share his fragmented research he had uncovered about the Oracle. He wished he had more information on the kids who were at the compound.

* * *

Samuel had spent the better part of an hour from 4:00 A.M. to the present locating a charter to fly him from Boise to San Francisco. It was the holiday weekend, though it was the day after Thanksgiving. Finally, he was able to hire a small Lear to whisk him to Katherine. The urgency seemed evident to Paul Hill as he taxied the chartered jet to Boise's main runway where he awaited tower approval to zoom into the sky with his one passenger, Samuel Meyers, in the cockpit beside him.

Earlier, Samuel had interrupted the family gathering.

It had been a tense scene, especially when Lance confronted him about traipsing off to San Francisco.

"So, Dad, you really think this is right?" Samuel's eldest son Lance had asked with a low voice. His light beard and unwashed face gave him a lumberjack look. The reddish, thin, curly hair had not even been combed. He had slipped on his trousers, thrown on a sweat shirt and was down stairs to drive Samuel to the airport before Samuel could call a taxi. It was 6:30 in the morning and Samuel wanted to get to the airport at 7:00. Paul Hill would be waiting at the southwest terminal where private planes were berthed at the commercial airport.

Lance could not resist cautioning his father about Katherine, even at this early hour. Samuel glanced over at his son with those blue eyes that were two shades darker than his own, friendly eyes , the eyes of a child and with assurance in his voice replied, "It's right. But don't worry, Son. I will not marry Katherine unless I can take her to the temple."

That had been all Lance wanted to hear. His early-morning face lit up. He reached over and patted him on the shoulder, and purred, "Dad, did I ever tell you how much you mean to me? You're the greatest. Really you are." He drove past the gate guard, directly to the aircraft whose engines were already humming. Samuel nearly leaped from the car.

Katherine had been up for an hour. She had never been an early riser, but lately it seemed she had difficulty sleeping past 7 in the morning. It was a little after 6 and here she was wide awake. She had been lying in bed for over half an hour trying to piece things together. With her robe on she wandered aimlessly into the kitchen and set the coffee maker. She had reduced her intake of coffee by half since she met Samuel and now strictly de-caf was all she would drink. She guessed that before long she might even give up the de-caf. Why worry now? Samuel's ever-so-slight disapproval would not be there. She could go back to full-strength coffee. Did it matter anymore? Really, did anything matter anymore?

Her mind suddenly reverted back to the thought that haunted her. If you love him so much then why worry whether you really believe in his faith? Go along with whatever they ask, to simply become a member of the Mormon Church. Just tell Samuel, just explain that we can have a wonderful life together. Does it really matter whether I truly believe in the Gospel of Christ as you do? Does it?

Katherine decided to take a frank look at her situation. If there is anything in my life that I can proudly point to, it's honesty. I have always been honest. With Bob, I went along with his religion because it was not an issue. I wanted him. He didn't care what I believed. He wanted me. It was really that simple.

Samuel is different. Very different. He is not demanding anything of me, but he wants me to be sincere in whatever I do. I can't do this to Samuel. I can't simply say I believe and lie. I can't.

She left the perking coffee maker and strolled into the living room. Through the floor-to-ceiling window she could see that the city was socked in; even before daylight the mist had swirled around the high-rise, sending rivulets of moisture down the glass obstructing even a clear view of the fog. It didn't matter. Katherine's heart was as filled with gloom as the gray mist pressing against the glass. A chill came over her. She stepped to the side of the veined fireplace and clicked the automatic lighter that created immediate blue and orange flames along the face of the stone logs.

That felt better.

She sat down on the facing sofa. Other than the fire, the only other light seeped in from the outside, and precious little of that, yet the glow of fluorescent bulbs cast their white light from the open door of the kitchen. She wanted it semi-dark, and wished she had closed the kitchen door on her way to the living room. The intense light shot diagonally across the dining room and cast its glow across the floor. She didn't want to get up off the couch and close the door; she would do that as soon as the coffee was ready.

Her mind retraced the last twenty-four hours. She didn't want to understand, but she knew deep in her soul that Samuel's family was right. They had religious commitments, and Samuel had loyalty to those he loved dearest. Why should he compromise for romantic love? Besides, Katherine felt she could never measure up to Samuel's first wife. From all she had heard about Margaret from the children, she had to have been a saint. What had she done with her life? *I'm selfish, worldly, love dresses and jewelry, money, position. Have I ever gone out of my way to truly help someone else? Never. Yet, why does Anney think I'm such a good person?*

Katherine smiled at the fire as she rehearsed Anney's outrage when she called her late last night. Still, Katherine boarded the flight, and now what? One lonely old lady seated in her penthouse, surrounded by material things. Nothing human to fill her empty heart. Once or twice she had prayed with Samuel. Granted, it was with the others before a trip, but they had bowed their heads together. Katherine felt good about Samuel's prayers. She never felt that he did it for show. Samuel's God listened to him. Katherine wondered aloud, "Where is my God. . . . God, I'm no Samuel, but I believe Samuel when he tells me you listen to his words. Am I so far from you that you can't hear my words —or you won't? Do you ever hear a plea from someone like me? Please, please. What am I to do? What is to become of me? Why can't I have your Samuel? He is a good man. I know I don't deserve him, but I so want him . What do I have to do to have this wonderful soul back in my life? God, are you hearing me? Samuel says if I pray sincerely you will listen. How much more sincere can I be? I want your Samuel. I need him."

It was nearly half an hour later before Katherine stepped back into the kitchen and poured her cup of de-caf, then carried it to her marble bathroom off the master bedroom where she would take over an hour to arrange her bone-thin, handsome face for the day. *Will he listen to me if I call him?* she wondered. She decided not to. Why? What would she say? She paused to see her reflection in the eight-foot-wide mirror. Glancing at herself in the glass, she pulled at her cheeks, then pinched the flesh between her eyes, causing the skin to wrinkle. She wondered why she even cared about her appearance if the one she loved had gone. Standing there, not entirely satisfied with her appearance, she made a little mental vow to top off the jilted feeling. *Monday morning, I'm going away. Far away where I can sort things out and come to my senses. Have*

_I been foolish. How could I expect someone like Samuel to love me? I must having been stupid to ever think he could. Yet . . ._

\* \* \*

"It could take us a few minutes. This has been a rushed affair, logging my flight plan, pulling the plane out of the hangar and now the tower has complete control of our take-off. We'll have to idle here a few minutes. The commercials have priority. They have schedules to keep. It won't be long, Sir."

Even five minutes perched to ascend into the sky was too long for Samuel. He had to share his inspired insight with Katherine and explain the vision he had seen, with her in person. The phone would never do. In spite of his unease at waiting to take off, he felt great comfort in what had been revealed to him. What a glorious night it had been, spoiled only by the fact that Katherine could not be told immediately. How would she respond to this latest revelation in his life? It affected her as much as him, but he had to explain it with the right tone, the right spirit.

Samuel knew that Katherine and he had a compelling love, but there were family, church, and tradition to consider. It had come to him in that dream that Katherine had not been fully awakened to the spirit of testimony. Good relationships, as well as seemingly good marriages, fail if they have only two of the three essentials of involvement, commitment, and respect. Katherine's spirit had to awaken. She didn't know what it was like to hunger and thirst after righteousness.

_Will she listen to me? Will Katherine come around? All I can do is hope and pray that she will accept the revelation as true._

"The tower says we're cleared for take off. You know it's less than an hour in this marvelous craft."

Samuel looked out the side window as the Lear taxied to the painted markings on the tarmac. His spirits soared as the Lear leaped forward. _Katherine._ Samuel felt he had experienced a night vision, one that he felt was intended not only for him, but Katherine as well. He had to tell her that he had approval from Margaret to seek after this good woman who had left so abruptly.

\* \* \*

Burton slept in. He was exhausted with all he had been doing for the past forty-eight hours or more. It was late afternoon when he awoke and the first thing he did was call Stephen and learned from Anney that Stephen had taken the boys to dinner and would be back later. He next tried to reach Samuel in Boise, then San Francisco.

\* \* \*

Dr. Mucranski smoothed out the faxed photo from the Thorns. She studied Brenda's large eyes and warm smile. Her beauty came through even on the somewhat distorted fax page. She had taken it to have Daniel study the face to determine  if he had seen Brenda before. "Did you ever see this girl at Gateway?" Dr. Mucranski asked casually, as if Daniel had met her at a debutante ball. It was, after all, a fax and therefore not a clear reproduction of the photo. The doctor wondered whether he would actually recognize the face. There were a lot of kids at the compound.

Daniel had gained confidence  in Dr. Mucranski. She had become his friend, his ally and main avenue to a sane world. He was willing to divulge whatever information he had to this kind person with an accent. He took one glance at the faxed photo and said as he held it in his right hand, "It's Rachel. I would know her face anywhere. It's her."

"You mean you saw this young lady in the compound?"

"Yes, she has been in the induction center inside the cave for a few weeks now. It's Rachel."

"Daniel, this girl's name is not Rachel; it is Brenda."

"Well, it's Rachel at Gateway. Yes, it's Rachel. I know her."

Dr. Mucranski was convinced it was the Thorn's daughter. That was the important thing.

# Chapter 19

It was midmorning Friday in San Francisco and Samuel didn't have to lodge his foot in the door. When Katherine saw who it was, she opened the door wide and fell into his arms, crying with pent-up emotion. They clung to each other, Samuel caressing her hair, rocking her slowly in his arms as she quietly sobbed. "Oh Samuel, how I prayed to God that I wouldn't lose you."

At last they loosened their hold and smiled shyly at each other. "Katherine, my sweet love," Samuel breathed, "we can surely figure this out. Anything worthwhile is worth working for. Will you at least talk to me about it?"

Katherine was on her own turf, and what a difference it made in her perspective. All she knew was that, regardless of family and religion, she wanted Samuel. He had filled her life with warmth and light, and without him, grayness and gloom took over.

Samuel plunged ahead in his explanation of why his children felt the way they did about the two of them and why he had not taken up the sword and slain all the dragons in his damsel's way. There were logical reasons for their reactions to Samuel's involvement with Katherine. They weren't simply defending home and hearth in remembrance of mother. In reality, their feelings for their mother had nothing to do with their reaction to father dating another woman. They wanted him to marry again; all had tried to convince him that he needed a loving companion. Samuel explained once again that it had everything to do with Katherine becoming a member of the Church and being worthy to marry in the temple.

His voice dropped to a near whisper. They were arm-in-arm on the sofa in the living room with the entire bay now stretched out before them now that the fog had lifted. The window poured morning light into the room.

He felt that the moment was right. He released himself from Katherine and turned his upper body in her direction. With a serious expression enveloping his features, he said, "Something happened to me after you left: Brad and I talked.

He told me you said that you believed in me. He said it happened while we were filming in Missouri. Is that right?"

"Yes, I told him that. I believe it. Really, I believe that you know where you're going. You know things about life and eternity that I don't. I really believe you know for certain that God will take us to Him. You have a conviction that I want. But, Samuel, I can't deceive you. I do not have the firm belief that you have, yet. . . . I may never have it. But I want to believe. I'm sure you know that I do." Katherine lowered her head.

Samuel looked down on her styled, light-gray hair. He felt a tenderness for this woman of honesty and strength. He knew that she did not have to have a testimony by the Spirit to believe in God's servants. The scriptures were very clear that some would not be blessed with the Spirit to have a personal witness; some would be taken to Christ by the testimony of others. Brad was right: Katherine had a testimony, the testimony of Samuel. "I believe you are my guide. I want to believe, Samuel, I truly do. Help me."

"I will, Katherine. I will. Though there is one thing you should know, and once again I'm pressing you to believe me. I'll go into detail later, still you need to know that my first wife Margaret came to me in a dream and told me that she approved of you as my wife. As I said you have to trust me on this one."

Close to Samuel's left ear, lips touching his neck, she whispered, "I know you are right. I just know it, my love."

He folded her closer into his arms and kissed her cheek. She pulled back, looked at him in the face and cupped her hands to his cheeks. "Are you telling me that this Holy Spirit is giving me the same conviction you have about the Church?"

"Yes, yes, yes. Katherine, it is only a beginning. But what a beginning."

"But it is a beginning." She repeated, "Trust me Samuel. I won't let this moment pass. I prayed right here, when I got up this morning, that God would help me. He has." Katherine shook her head from side-to-side in wonder. "I'll hang on. I will, Samuel. I surely will."

When Samuel and Katherine picked up their luggage at the Salt Lake airport, Stephen was standing nearby listening to Samuel explain all about the complexities of Thanksgiving with the family, Katherine's flight and his chase to appease her in San Francisco. Stephen listened as Samuel explained and Katherine filled in some of the details, all in a rush of words. Stephen's only comment was "Yeah, I heard a little about it from Anney after you called her from the airport in Boise, Katherine. Things okay now?"

"Yes. I think so. How is Anney?" Katherine asked with a tone of voice that meant she wanted the straight scoop. "Did she actually think she could get into that place up in Jackson Hole and get Brenda out? She didn't even know for sure that Brenda was there."

"She told you, did she?"

Katherine's eyes revealed all.

"She's okay," Stephen said, "Just one real stressed-out woman. Once she got over the euphoria of knowing that Brenda was at Gateway. Now, reality set in and she is still distressed that something may happen up there."

"Well, you can't blame her for that." Samuel could sense that Stephen was not going to go into detail. "So we're pretty certain that Brenda is at the hellhole in Wyoming?"

"I'm convinced she's there, and the authorities believe she is."

"Well let's get her out," Katherine said. She was a woman whose demands were met regularly.

Stephen helped Samuel toss his large bag on a cart and started for the elevator to the parking terrace. "That is exactly what we are going to do. Anney is at home putting things together. We're going up to Jackson as soon as possible."

"By the way, where's Burton now?" Samuel asked.

"He should be at my place pretty soon. He said he was driving down from here so we could all meet at my place."

\* \* \*

Thom Burton was there. He had spent the day continuing his research on the Oracle, then he had rushed down from Salt Lake City to be on hand at Stephen's and Anney's home. He arrived ten minutes before the three arrived from the airport.

They had all come together for a briefing and to make a decision on where they stood in relationship to the pressing problem of freeing Brenda.

It was dark by five-fifteen. Anney came into the family room and switched on the lamps, asking Thom if she could sit in on the discussion. She was not certain what was happening, but the gathering gave her hope. At least things were beginning to shape into a first-rate investigation.

"Thom, you've been in contact with the FBI and the sheriff. What's happening?" Anney began.

"They're pulling together every shred of evidence possible. Believe me, Mrs. Thorn . . . "

"Call me Anney."

"Okay, Anney, they want to put this Oracle guy away if they can. They need to line up their case and that's what they're doing. They won't act until they are sure they have enough to put him and those who are working with him away." He was impressed with this woman. He had only met her a couple of days ago, but felt that he knew her.

There was a sense of urgency to the meeting. Things had been happening rapidly. The FBI had confirmed Daniel's recognition of Brenda in the photo and was ready to move. Burton had in turn received calls from the sheriff wanting to know everything he knew about the sudden death of Roy, since he was the last to see him alive.

Burton felt the time was right to lay out all he had researched on the Oracle and the situation in Wyoming. "I couldn't bring myself to tell you earlier all that I've learned about the Oracle." His eyes moved from Anney to Stephen and back to Anney. "I don't know that it's all true, but if it is, then the authorities have to think very carefully about how they will go about smoking this guy out. Matter of fact, we don't even know that he's at the compound. Rumor has it that he is building a smaller but basically similar compound in Central America. The sheriff, however, seems pretty certain that the guy is still inside the compound. You know we're looking at a rather fortified place. From what Dr. Mucranski has learned from Daniel, there is a large cave to the east of the main building. Who knows what that idiot Oracle has stashed away inside there."

"What do you mean a 'cave, and stuff stashed away?'" Anney asked. Her mouth had a dour expression. She felt her skin freeze. This was news to the others as well, but Anney's reaction was intense.

Burton drew breath and continued to explain what he had amassed in his investigation by talking to Dr. Mucranski and the sheriff, as well as some of his news sources in Wyoming, plus other newsmen on the coast, and as far away as Maryland where the Oracle grew up. He had a complete dossier on the Oracle. It was scary. Burton explained how the man had traveled throughout Asia and South America, acquainting himself with some of the most notorious individuals who claimed to be scientists or human experimenters on the globe.

When he dipped deeper into the sadistic character of the Oracle, according to his information, Burton couldn't help noticing that Anney had gone pale. Burton hesitated to go on with the Oracle's dossier. He shifted to a summary of what he felt the Oracle intended to do at Gateway. "I think the man is trying to create a group of people who will become totally subservient to his wishes."

"What is his ultimate goal?" Samuel asked.

"Oh, I think he feels that he is an instrument for God and that it is the wish of God to have his children be obedient to his will and to erase all human follies as we know them from the face of the earth."

"How does he think this is possible?" Stephen probed.

"I don't know the answer to that question."

"Have you told the sheriff in Jackson what you've discovered in your research?" Anney asked.

"Most of what I've learned I've shared with all the law enforcement people. I'm still piecing this together. What I know about this clown in Jackson, I've had to dig up in the past couple of days. It wasn't until I listened to what Dr. Mucranski knew about the Oracle and the information she shared with me about her interview with Daniel that I really started digging into this thing. I haven't confirmed any of my sources. Some of the findings may be out in left field. All I can say, off the record, is that we are dealing with a sick man, and I mean a real sicko."

For some strange reason, Anney's earlier fears while listening to Thom abated as she absorbed all that was tumbling out of his investigative report. Suddenly she was hungry for information, any information, no matter how hard to hear. She wanted action, and now. It was the sheer knowledge that something was being done that lifted her spirits.

"What can we do?" Stephen asked, hoping that Burton, with all of his information, would have some solution to the problem of getting Brenda out of there and safely home.

"Isn't this the reason we are here this evening? We need to come up with a plan. We need to take action."

Samuel voiced his concern. "I still think we ought to get on the phone with the federal authorities and let them know we want to help in any way possible. They have to be the ones to take action."

"That sounds well and good, but I don't think they will act. Okay?" Burton snapped.

"Why?" Samuel said, noting a tension in Burton's tone that was unusual for the man. He had seemed almost detached up to this point.

Stephen looked at Anney, transmitting in their private code a question she immediately understood. Stephen was asking, *What's with this guy? He needs to chill out.* Her response, equally silent, was, *Hold on. Let's hear him out.*

"What are you talking about?" Samuel persisted, unmoved by Burton's rebuff. "Why can't we put pressure on the authorities to act?" Samuel had the stuff that Katherine found appealing and masculine. He stood up to those around him.

"I'll tell you why." Burton came up from the cream-colored leather chair and pointed his finger at Samuel, hunching his shoulders, preparing to do battle. "You wanna know why? Because this guy Josiah, the great Oracle, is a Hitler. Did you know that Hitler devised a program from his bunker, where he was forced to retreat near the end . . . a program to destroy all the major cities in Europe? He commanded his military leaders to burn all cities behind them. 'Level them!' he told his subordinates. Some did and some didn't. Warsaw got it, as did a number of cities in Poland. The Oracle will destroy everything and everybody if he's pressed to the wall."

"He's right, Stephen," Anney said wide-eyed. "I read about it last year while we were in Europe with Daddy. Hitler did destroy their cities. What a cruel thing at the end of the war."

"She's got that right," Burton said, turning his index finger in Anney's direction. "From what this Daniel has told Dr. Mucranski, the Oracle plans to do the same thing. There are explosives situated at strategic points around the compound. If any of the authorities try to storm the place, he'll set off the explosives. He's crazy. He's as nuts as any cult leader we've dealt with in the past two decades or more. The guy is ready for the jacket. He is really dangerous. I didn't tell you earlier because I didn't want to frighten you."

"Well, you've done a good job now," Katherine muttered.

Burton continued, "We all know that, based on what has been uncovered to this point, Roy was a victim of this madman. Our problem is that we can't prove it." Stephen raised his voice as he spoke. "Roy must have known something incriminating about them, so they silenced him and burned the Center. I have no doubt any longer that he was a victim of the Oracle's madness."

"Action is what is needed," Samuel insisted. "I think a couple of us need to go up to Jackson Hole and try to piece this whole thing together with the authorities. And maybe take some action."

"Action? What action? I agree, but what can we do?" Stephen demanded of Burton. "All I know is that as a distressed father I can't just sit around and wait for something to happen. I want to cause something to happen."

Samuel cautioned, "It might be a little premature for us to do something on our own that we will regret. Let's wait a day or two and see what more Dr. Mucranski can pry out of Daniel. Timing is an important factor in this whole mess. I say we wait a while longer."

"I agree with waiting a couple of days, but after that, something has to be done." Burton nodded. "But we have to keep up the pressure all around. I'll finish my report in the morning and fax it to both the FBI agent and Sheriff Harmon. I would think that the FBI has already done a thorough study of the Oracle and realizes what he's up to, but it can't hurt for me to communicate with them. What I have is mostly from talk among journalists. It is not the sort of thing you can use to invade the compound."

\* \* \*

Sheriff Harmon sat in the same row with Massey, one seat dividing them. The flight out of Santa Fe was only a third filled. They had endured a long day of travel and investigation and now they would be late getting back to Jackson Hole. Massey looked searchingly into Harmon's interested face. "I'm ready to move on this Oracle, but we need to line up all of the evidence." Massey had called the director in Washington while at the airport in Santa Fe shortly before boarding the plane. "My boss has given me full authority to act on this whole matter, when I feel ready. You know, we've been investigating the Oracle for some time. He's slippery, but there is no question that the guy is dirty. The only concern my boss has is the way we go about it. He will give me over a hundred men from all over the West if I need them to go into Gateway and make arrests. Horn, we need more proof that he has in fact violated federal law. Did he cross over state lines to commit crimes? Does he in fact have illegal military weapons at the compound? Do we have enough proof that he in fact has committed murder inside that compound? We need more witnesses. If I could get one more piece of solid evidence  that he has illegal weapons or whatever, I'd be inside that compound in a New York minute."

"What about the explosives this madman can set off? We're all convinced he has them stashed around the place."

"We may be able to work it out without it coming to such an insane conclusion."

"From what I'm hearing, you and your people will run the show if it comes to moving in force. Is that right?"

"Right. But I will still need your help. You know the area. You can do a great deal with access, lookouts, and advise me on the best approach. It may be shaping up into a federal case, but I'll need you close at hand."

"Oh, don't worry, I'll be available with my people to help every way I can."

"Good."

# Chapter 20

He knew it was a long shot, but worth testing. The meeting at the Thorns' had just concluded. Thom felt confused. Things were not in their hands, anyway. The authorities had complete control. He pondered what they had discussed this evening and could come to no resolution as he sped along University Avenue in sparse traffic from the Thorns' home. He was headed south and not west to the freeway as normally he would have done. He felt the urge to follow up on an impression he had received when he started the engine of his car.

He made a left at the signal light, but hadn't a clue as to why he felt compelled to swing by the burned-out shell of the Book of Mormon Center before heading for the freeway and his apartment in Salt Lake City. He circled the block where the Center had stood, looking out the passenger side of his car into the faint light from the street lamps. He could hardly make out the twisted steel beams and black remains of the Center. On the second pass he nosed his car into the entrance ramp and stopped short of a six-foot-high temporary wire fence that had been thrown up the day after the fire. No one was allowed access to the parking lot east of the ashes. He didn't care. It was not his intent to go beyond the wire fencing. He got out and walked along the sidewalk to where the side wall of the Center had stood. He strained his vision, trying to make out the ruins twenty feet from the sidewalk. He thought of Roy and could almost reenact the scene of horror as the building went up in flames.

Burton had been to the fire-gutted building twice before, but tonight he felt a strange compulsion to view it once again. Why, he didn't know. The group session at the Thorns' had lasted until 11:00 p.m. He needed sleep and home was a good hour up the freeway, but still he felt he *had* to make another visual inspection of the Center.

Thoughts jostled about inside his head. He let his mind rove over those two days he had spent with Roy in Jackson Hole. He forced his thoughts to recall every detail of those days. *Did Roy act out of the ordinary? What have*

*I overlooked that seems to be gnawing at me? What exactly did Roy say or do to signal his distress?*

Thom recalled the bus ride from Jackson to Salt Lake City and remembered that Roy had typed notes on his laptop as the bus sped along the highway from Jackson on that return trip. Thom allowed his mind to recreate that scene. He recalled nothing out of the ordinary as he flashed those memories across his mind, hoping to detect the least little tidbit. At that point in his travels with Roy, Burton remembered that he knew nothing about Daniel. Yet Roy had met Daniel in the compound, according to information from New Mexico.

Suddenly, voicing his frustration out loud, Burton said, "Roy, why didn't you confide in me on the bus? I wanted to help you and set your mind at ease. Why? Why?" Suddenly, Burton's own thoughts startled him. The name "Daniel" came into focus as if he heard Roy's voice, as if someone had spoken the words to him. *Try the name Daniel.*

Strange. The name Daniel seemed to glow in his thoughts. Then it came to him. *Daniel. That's it. Could it be this simple? If there were hidden files, then the password could very well be Daniel. Did Roy stash his typed thoughts about what had happened at Gateway under the code name 'Daniel'? It was worth a try. All Burton needed at the moment was Roy's laptop.*

He and Stephen had been over that path once before without success. There was nothing out of the ordinary on the main file or the disk Roy worked from when they checked it out days ago. *But what if all they lacked was the password?* The more Burton rolled the thought around in his mind, the more convinced he became that he had to at least try the password "Daniel." He would do it tonight! He hit the wire fence with the palms of his hands, excited to try. He was onto something. He hoped the Thorns were not in bed. Stephen had told Burton just yesterday on the phone that he intended to turn over Roy's electronic equipment to the Provo police investigative team. He hadn't. It was still at the Thorns', along with all the other electronic equipment removed from Roy's apartment and tagged to be shipped ultimately to Roy's family in Boston.

Burton took a final glance at the ghost-like ruins of the Center, then whirled about and rushed to his car. "I hate to do this to you, Stephen," Burton mouthed out loud, "but I have to take a look at that laptop right now."

Burton pounded on Stephen's front door. It was nearing midnight. Stephen and Anney had not yet fallen asleep. The noise of Burton's knock startled them.

"Who could that be?" Anney asked, troubled at any sound.

"I'll look. You stay put," Stephen said, crawling out of bed. He tossed on his robe and groped for his slippers in the dark to avoid shining the bright bedroom light in Anney's eyes. He hurried out of the bedroom to the front door barefoot.

Anney had no intentions of staying in bed. As Stephen disappeared in the dark, she turned over and switched on the lamp on her side of the bed. Whoever it was seemed insistent and that meant something had happened. She wanted to know. Out of bed, she grabbed her peach-colored robe and slippers and rushed after Stephen. In the hall she heard Stephen open the front door and say, "Thom!"

By the time Anney was halfway across the dark living room with faint light from the night light in the entrance hall, Thom was in the house, closing the door behind him.

"Sorry, really I am," Thom apologized in his smooth form, though the words were clipped. "It's late, but I have an idea about the password to Roy's laptop. The one he was typing on in the bus that night. Can we haul it out and test my theory?"

Stephen wanted to say that Burton had better be right. It was late, and they had a full day ahead of them. He and Burton had compared notes repeatedly over the last few days, trying to discover the file that Burton insisted Roy must have composed and saved. It would have been out of character for Roy to have typed material on the bus and not saved it.

It took Burton all of one minute once he had the laptop on, to access the coded file. While the Toshiba booted up, Burton glanced up at Stephen and in an excited tone of voice, said, "The password is Daniel. Wait and see if I'm not right."

The screen lit up, Burton typed in "Daniel" and waited a second. Scarcely breathing, the three stood looking into the monitor, when a text suddenly flashed on the screen. Burton read aloud what Roy had written:

"I AM MAKING THESE NOTES SO I WILL CLEARLY RECALL WHAT I OVERHEARD YESTERDAY AFTERNOON. I OVERHEARD THE ORACLE AND HIS CHIEF OF SECURITY, REUBEN, DISCUSS THE ASSIGNED KILLING OF SETH, A YOUNG MAN HERE IN THE COMPOUND. THEY SPOKE OF TAKING HIS BODY TO THE SLOPES AND MAKING IT LOOK LIKE THE YOUNG MAN

HAD BEEN KILLED IN A JEEP ACCIDENT WHEN THE VEHICLE WENT OVER THE SIDE AND CRASHED INTO THE ROCKS BELOW. I HAVE TRIED TO PUSH THIS FROM MY MIND SINCE I FIRST OVERHEARD THEM TALKING IN THE REST ROOM. (THEY DIDN'T KNOW I WAS IN THE ENCLOSED STALL.) I THINK THEY SUSPECT SOMETHING. THEY TRIED TO REMOVE ME FROM THE BUS WHILE WE WERE EXITING THE FRONT GATE. I FEEL THAT MY LIFE IS IN DANGER. . . . I SHOULD HAVE KNOWN THEY HAD CAMERA SURVEILLANCE. I KNEW THEY MUST HAVE SEEN ME WHEN THEY CAME TO TAKE ME OFF THE BUS.

The note ended as if Roy had wanted to explain more, but felt compelled to save the notes and place them on the main file as coded material.

"They killed him," Stephen said with one hand out, palm flat, his jaw set in anger.

"Yep, they sure as hell did," Burton growled. His shoulders slumped and he wore a disheartened expression. "I didn't know the guy that well. But looking back, I can see I should have probed more while we were on the bus. We could have gone to the police in Salt Lake that very night. I just didn't measure up. I sensed that he might be in jeopardy, but I did nothing about it."

Anney touched Burton's slack shoulder and whispered, "Thom, don't beat yourself up. How could you know? How could any of us know?"

Anney, the practical one at the moment, turned to Stephen with a beam of understanding. She, too, felt like she was experiencing the news of Roy's death all over again, but she had control of her emotions and said slowly, "You know what this means? That file on his notebook computer is dated. This is evidence that Roy was murdered. This will give the FBI the means to smoke out that damnable man at Gateway."

The three stood over the monitor a while longer, hashing over the details of what they should do with the new-found evidence. Stephen suggested they fax a copy of the document to the sheriff's office immediately. Burton cautioned against that. He was still afraid that someone in the sheriff's office might give the Oracle the information. "You print it out, Stephen. Then we'll take the laptop and pull it up in the sheriff's presence." Burton was nearly breathless. "We've got to get up there to Jackson."

"Okay, but not until morning. No one is going to do anything during the night," Stephen reasoned. He knew Anney would leave within the hour if he said the word.

Burton stepped back, and Anney and Stephen debated the idea of leaving for Jackson first thing in the morning. They reasoned that they would have to notify Samuel and that he would want to pick up Katherine before leaving. "Okay, then," Stephen concluded. "We'll leave at 8:00 in the morning. We'll camp out at one of the motels if we have to, but the authorities are going to know that we mean to get this thing resolved once and for all."

It was after 2:00 in the morning. Burton had left. Anney had finally dropped off to sleep, only to be jarred awake after a few moments. When she rolled over, she sensed that Stephen was not on his side of the big bed. She could see in the dim light that the bathroom door was open and no one was in there. Groggy but alarmed, she rolled out of bed and walked out of the bedroom. She slipped through the hall that was illuminated by a night light plugged in near the floor. She looked into the living room, then walked to the kitchen. No Stephen. From the kitchen she could see the flickering light of the television screen aglow in the family room. When she entered the room, she saw Stephen's head leaning back on the sofa as he watched the images of their children at play. She stood for a moment silently watching six-year-old Brenda rush up to the video camera and stick out her tongue playfully. Anney remembered the day: It was the 4th of July, and the whole family was having a barbecue in their backyard in Lafayette.

Tears welled up in her eyes as she watched the video camera focus on little Brenda, detailing her every move: her smile, her white teeth, her bright eyes so full of wonder and happiness. It was almost more than Anney could stand. Up to now, she had purposely not reviewed the family films since Brenda left college early. She knew she would fall apart.

Still silent, she moved in behind Stephen and dropped her arms around his neck from behind the sofa. Her touch startled him. He jerked his head around to see who it was. There was a broad question in his face as he looked at Anney. Then she saw the tears cascading down his cheeks. She wanted to ask him why he was torturing himself, but the words wouldn't form. She simply leaned down and kissed his cheek and pressed her face next to his. She knew he was as tormented by this situation with Brenda as she.

Stephen finally clicked off the VCR and stood up. Paramount in his mind were all the ways things could go sour in Jackson Hole. He wouldn't mention them. Not tonight. Anney needed to remain as emotionally stable as possible, and it was his duty to see to that. "We both have to get some sleep, honey. Tomorrow is already here, and we will soon have some traveling to do."

# Chapter 21

The Thorns' Jeep was packed. It was Saturday morning, still considered part of the Thanksgiving weekend. It seemed to Anney they had crammed a year's concern into the past three days. She stuffed her down pillow into a narrow space behind the rear seat as Stephen slammed the tailgate down on the bulging Grand Cherokee. Samuel had pulled his Buick up behind Stephen's Jeep and tossed two remaining bags in the trunk. It was decided that Todd would drive the Thorns' car, with Max as shotgun and Katherine and Anney in the rear of the Jeep. Stephen had already indicated that part of the way to Jackson Hole he needed to discuss business with Samuel, and asked if anyone would mind if he and Samuel drove alone at least for the first hour and a half, then maybe switch places. Everyone agreed.

Set to pull out, Anney sensed that something unpleasant would happen once they got to Gateway. Yet, somehow, some way, they would get Brenda out. Anney had already vowed to herself that she was not coming back without her daughter. Stephen walked back into the house to get Roy's laptop that he had carefully packed into a box with Styrofoam peanuts to cushion it.

There was a sense of adventure in the air. Anney couldn't altogether comprehend why she felt so excited and concerned at the same time. "Maybe," she had said to Stephen while packing, "it has to do with a positive feeling that one way or another we're going to get our Brenda. We are, you know."

\* \* \*

By mid-afternoon Martha left Reuben with his beer at the bar and walked with deliberate steps to the double doors of the Wild Horse Saloon. There was apprehension in her eyes as she strolled outside, making every effort possible to remain calm. In front of the bar the sidewalk was constructed of wooden planks that reverberated with the sounds of dozens of boots clipping along as tourists invaded the town. She could feel her pulse throbbing in her temples.

Sweat was forming on her brow. She noticed that the tourists were out in numbers. Good, they would offer cover.

Martha had made final arrangements the day before. The decision to leave the compound had come gradually over the last few weeks. Now that she was acting on that decision, she realized that she would rather spend time in prison than remain another day at Gateway at the mercy of the Oracle. There was a chance that if she worked her cards right, she would get a lighter sentence by cooperating with the authorities about what she knew was happening at the compound and the military weapons hidden there. It was her only hope.

Actually, she had decided to leave the compound the night she learned about Dr. Chang and his team of two other surgeons who were coming to experiment on two of the compound members. Did it matter that one of those two happened to be Rachel? She only knew that a transformation had taken place inside her head. Exactly why her attitude had changed, she could only guess. But she knew that the Oracle's appalling plan to clone humans was a major factor in her decision to cut and run.

For an instant in the naked sunlight of downtown Jackson, Martha panicked and almost retraced her steps to the Wild Horse to rejoin Reuben and return to what had been a safe haven inside the compound; then she took a mental grip on her emotions and kept walking to her destination up the street. She tried to melt into the crowd, steeling her nerves to go through with her plan of escape from hell.

Martha had spent the last few weeks trying to come to grips with her troubling thoughts and assemble the bits and pieces of her life. Over and over she thought, *Who am I to make a judgment call on the Oracle's new direction to set up a perfect society?* After all, hadn't she assisted him in every way in altering the minds of the young people at Gateway? She had participated in her assigned work up to the very moment she left the cave just hours ago, yet somehow her own methods seemed less reprehensible than cloning.

Something—what it was, she could not pinpoint—something in her rebelled against participating in cloning and implanting chips to make robotic figures. That night when she left the Oracle's office, she had searched the Net in the communications center. Jeremiah had even assisted her on the search engines to locate the latest discussions on cloning. She had seen that there were dozens of people and media organizations flooding the Web site with comments and scientific news on cloning. One guy, she recalled, had asked the question, " . . . What makes me me, and you?" Then he had answered his own question: "I know we are more than cells strung together to form a shell we call a body. There is more, much more. Our memories, emotions of love and hate. I'm sorry, but there is more to us than merely cells grouped together."

She had already reasoned out in her mind that life cannot exist without a soul. So, if a clone were to live, it would have a soul. Then late that night, studying the comments on the Web sites, she had come to realize that vast scientific possibilities and ethical dilemmas were growing to gigantic proportions on this issue of genetic human engineering. She could also see that bioethical issues meant nothing to the Oracle. Why had that surprised her? Not for a long time had she felt such hatred for any person as she did at this moment of escape for the Oracle. She had to get to the authorities . . . she *had* to. If the Oracle went unchecked, some of the compound members would suffer irreversible life changes.

Over a week before, Martha had taken careful steps that set her escape plans into motion. It was the Teton Purity Water service attendant that sealed the deal for her escape. Martha had developed a relationship with the older fellow who came each week to exchange the water in Josiah's private indoor pool. For two years Martha had greeted Charley and talked of little more than water and daily life, but in the process, Charley had revealed his lifestyle. He told Martha more than once that his wife was too fat, that he loved fishing, hiking in the Tetons in the summertime, and planned to retire in three more years. All of these tidbits of ordinary life with a straight person from the outside tugged at Martha's desire for such a life. She began to long for the life of Charley's wife. Nothing special. Over the two years of meeting Charley at the pool, she had come to trust him.

When Martha whispered to Charley that she planned to escape the compound, she had asked him to find an attorney for her to meet with, someone Charley trusted. He suggested George Wilkins. Martha knew better than to simply walk in cold to the sheriff's office and try to cut a deal. She needed professional advice to make such an enormous step. Her very freedom in the future depended on the skill of the attorney. Martha was well aware that she was relying on Charley to get her the best lawyer for her case. She had no other choice.

The letter from Martha to George Wilkins, which she slipped to Charley beside the pool, asked him to meet her a block from the Wild Horse Saloon at 3:30 this afternoon. When she slipped the letter to Charley, their backs to the monitors in the pool room, he described George to her. No one had noticed anything unusual, since Martha always helped him with the hose that extended to the bottom of the Oracle's pool.

It was set. George agreed to wear a green woolen scarf and white cowboy hat and meet her a block from the Wild Horse Saloon. She spotted him half a block away, and trying not to appear eager, she moved with a steady pace to his side. Charley had told her he was in his sixties, tall, and wrinkled in the face. The description fit. When she stood beside him on the plank sidewalk, Martha refused to make eye contact with George. With a deadpan expression, her voice strangely flat, as if all emotion had been drained from her, she said, "I'm Martha. Can we go somewhere and talk?"

"To my office," George said in a voice nearly as deadpan as Martha's.

* * *

The sheriff took the call in his office. His chair tilted back, he gazed at the far wall without seeing the two sets of mounted elk horns that had come with the seventy-year-old building. The room had been redecorated twice since it became the sheriff's office in the early 1970s, but the decorators had worked around the elk horns, keeping the dusty old relics the focal point of the room.

"Sheriff . . . "

"Yeah. Hey, George." Martha's new attorney had been friends with the sheriff for the past twenty years. They had been on good terms most of those years.

George went directly into the subject of one Martha—"Don't ask what her real name is; she went by the name of Martha in the compound."—who wanted to cut a deal with the sheriff. That was the starting point. It took George the better part of thirty minutes to swing a plea-bargain deal. The sheriff cautioned George that he was not a judge and anything he agreed to could and might be changed in a court of law. But if this Martha was willing to tell all, he would keep his end of the deal to protect her and urge the judge to be fair.

"Bring her in, George. This is our first real break with this Oracle fellow."

* * *

Reuben called Jeremiah from the executive suite as the assassin sat before the computer to see if Martha had checked in with him. She hadn't. He turned to look at the Oracle and said with a quiet, firm voice, "I have a good idea that Martha has skipped. I think she's at the bus depot. The next bus is due out in an hour. It was the first place I looked, but she could be hiding nearby, ready to run to the bus at the last minute."

"In other words, you're not sure just where she is at this time?" the Oracle said with a bitter, mocking tone in his voice.

"Well, no, but I think she's headed out of town."

* * *

The deputy sheriff positioned himself beside the wing of the commuter jet as five men from Seattle, all FBI, made their way down the stairs from the open door of the plane. They had come to Jackson Hole from their connecting flight at Boise. This was the fifth group of large, intelligent-looking fellows to step off commuters in the past eight hours. The airport officials allowed Deputy Sheriff Markworth to pull his car onto the tarmac in order to secretly shuttle the disembarking group to the sheriff's office in Jackson.

Light snowflakes had swept across the tarmac when Burton spotted the deputy as he drove out to the plane. Nothing subtle about the agents' arrivals, Burton thought. The deputy was dressed in a woolen uniform and a heavy trailblazer jacket with the collar pulled up around his ears. The icy wind of the early evening was biting at the top of his pink ears. He was a bulky man, somewhere in his fifties, Burton guessed, a seasoned officer of the law.

Burton ran to the driver's side of the deputy's car, and as the door opened he extended his right hand. The deputy emerged from his car before reluctantly taking Burton's hand. "Thom Burton. Sir, I heard that groups of FBI agents have been gathering here in Jackson Hole all day. May I ask you why?"

Deputy Sheriff Markworth was puzzled. He thought the wraps were still on as far as knowledge of the FBI assembling was concerned. He sensed Burton was a journalist. The cocky- voiced young man was too pushy and self-confident to be anything else.

\* \* \*

When the group arrived in Jackson Hole, they had met with the sheriff and the FBI man, Massey, where they turned over the laptop to the authorities, then asked the sheriff to pull up Roy's file and read all about a murder at Gateway. The response was one of caution. The sheriff thanked them for the information, then asked that the group remain in their motel, or at least not interfere with FBI plans to investigate the matter further. Purposely vague, Burton had explained to the group on the way back to their motel that it was standard procedure for law enforcement people to be secretive. But he intended to move around town and find out what, if anything, was being done to move on the Oracle and his compound. He had struck gold when he cornered a journalist at the local TV station and learned about the FBI men arriving by commuter jets, and not just a couple. It looked to be a major contingent of agents.

Now, Burton wanted to know from the deputy whether the FBI was acting on the evidence that had been turned over to them, or through their own investigation. He knew from what he learned that throughout the day agents had been arriving from points all over the West. He knew from experience that this meant a move against the Oracle. It had to be.

The deputy pulled a ring of keys from his side and fumbled them in both hands to find the key to the Buick. He tried to ignore Burton and spoke to the five agents, "My car's right over here." He pointed toward the Buick.

"Then you're not going to comment on why there are so many agents in town?"

"Look, fella," the deputy said, moving his head back and forth, "you know we can't let anything out about what the federal government plans to do. Don't stir up any trouble. This is a confidential gathering. Do you think Eisenhower said much about the Normandy invasion to the press before the ships started blasting the shoreline of Normandy? Let's leave it at that."

Burton couldn't have been more pleased that at last something was happening.

\* \* \*

The assignment was easy enough for Jeremiah, that is, if Martha was still in Jackson trying to leave town. He had warned her to make a clean, quick break if she was going to cut out. He never promised her that he would not hunt her down and take final action. He liked Martha, but the $25,000 the Oracle would pay to take her out made all the difference. He would treat it as a job, nothing personal. Maybe Martha would understand. He didn't care if she didn't.

How long had she been missing? Reuben last saw her at about four o'clock when she left the bar and didn't return to the pickup at six. It was now eight. They had checked the airport. No one matching her description had taken a flight out of town. The bus depot said the next bus for Salt Lake City was leaving at 9:10, and the last bus to leave town would depart at 2:00 in the morning. Jeremiah had already checked out the bus depot and the blocks surrounding it. No Martha. He reasoned to himself that she was still in town. She had no credit card; Jeremiah knew that from a conversation with her at the compound. They didn't fraternize all that much, but she was a female, still with some looks and interesting to listen to. Still in all, it would not be a strain to kill her; her life was behind her, anyway. What did she have to look forward to? Like Jeremiah, she would have to remain low profile and almost in total hiding the rest of her life. With her record, if they ever pulled her in for any reason and did a fingerprint check on her, she was doomed. But then so was he. He mentally went through his routine checklist: Do nothing stupid to warrant arrest; avoid the cops; avoid people, except for his quarry.

Jeremiah was beginning to experience that same creeping high that he had the night he tailed that gawky fellow down to Provo and snuffed out his lights. Strange. He began to hunger for the sight of Martha. He knew the Oracle would want her eliminated. That was his job, but how long before he would turn her over to the Oracle? A feeling of ecstasy shot its way from the pit of his stomach to the very tingling hair follicles in his scalp. This was sheer excitement. Nothing like it in all the world.

The pickup moved slowly from block to block. The streets had patchy sheets of ice that Jeremiah could feel in the play of the steering wheel. He had already engaged the four-wheel drive and the Ford pickup felt secure. Encased in the cab, he felt somewhat aloof from the hostile environment. Though the city had street lamps spaced fifty feet apart, people walking along the sidewalks were shadows, hard to define. He moved, slowing to the right as traffic buzzed past him. Jeremiah prided himself on his ability to spot his prey, even in the semi-darkness of street lamps. Martha would be somewhere on the street in the next few minutes, maybe moving from one store to the next in an effort to remain out of sight as much as possible. She would emerge. Jackson was a relatively small town, only about ten blocks in a cluster of crowded shops. He would ~~spot her. He felt~~ confident of it. He also surmised that she would, once confronted, get into the pickup at his insistence. She was not the type to scream and stir about in a fit of anger. She would resign herself to the doom that awaited her. Hadn't it been that way on two occasions in New York four years ago? Jeremiah understood the human mind. He sensed that Martha lacked fight to go on.

* * *

*She has to be on the street by now,* Jeremiah thought as he turned the corner and studied the pedestrians walking under the Western style overheads along the wooden sidewalk. *There!* In a ski jacket with the hood down, the long black hair and slender body had every appearance of Martha. She was walking alone with a large leather bag slung over her shoulder. He was moving past the pedestrian lane when he caught her within his peripheral vision. He decided to move ahead and make a U-turn at the intersection so he would be on her side of the street. He would pull in suddenly and confront her. It was always best to confront a scared person in a crowd. She would freeze in silence as he escorted her to the pickup, shove her in from the driver's side, climb in behind her, and take off. Jeremiah had his window down and his rear view mirror adjusted to see his prey on the left side of the street. Oh, she's going in to shop. He could not risk losing her. Maybe the shop was one of those mini malls. He had been to town only three times before. He never felt secure walking the streets of Jackson, regardless of the many tourists that could shield his true identity. He knew he was wanted in three states as well as by the Feds. Why chance it by strolling around town, and for what?

Wanting to accost Martha before she could disappear inside a series of shops, Jeremiah impulsively turned sharply to his left and made his U-turn midblock. He then glided the vehicle to the curb. He sat in the driver's seat focused on the back of the woman who was studying something in the display window of one of the Western shops. He was certain it was Martha. Typically, he thought, like so many females, she was admiring the window display of bronze and ceramic figures of horses, cowboys, and Indians all in array.

Jeremiah studied the scene for a moment. He knew mistakes came with haste. *Figure it out. Go slow.* He glanced to his right to calculate the crowd of tourists moving along the plank sidewalk. There were at least a dozen people ambling along amid outbursts of laughter. It was a typical Saturday evening in Jackson.

While his attention was fixed on the female at the display window, Jeremiah failed to see the patrol car pull up behind him and two officers step from the vehicle. One remained near the right door of the patrol car, while the younger, larger, swaggering officer approached Jeremiah's pickup.

Jeremiah had rolled up the window by the time he stopped near the curb to study the back of the woman he thought was Martha. When she at length turned to continue walking, Jeremiah could see by the aged face that it was not Martha. His heart sank. She had looked so much like Martha from the back. Now he had to continue his search. His stomach began to churn. It was that old hopeless emotion that had stymied him on more than one crime spree when the victim became difficult to kill. No longer did he have the high that had come over him fifteen minutes earlier. It was not going to be so simple after all.

Just then the young officer tapped the driver-side window of the pickup. Jeremiah had been looking to his right with the back of his head toward the window. He turned and lost his cool. He hesitated for a moment, wide eyed in spite of his long experience with sudden encounters. He had not thought a police officer would enter the arrangement. The officer motioned for Jeremiah to lower the window. There was only a brief hesitancy on the part of Jeremiah before complying with the request.

*Remain in control. Don't panic! You have a driver's license and the pickup is registered in a corporate name. Not to worry, not to worry.* He kept repeating this phrase in his mind as the officer spoke.

"Good evening, sir," the police officer said.

*They are all so courteous, all so pure and holy. I hate cops.*

"Are you aware that you made a U-turn in the middle of the block?"

Jeremiah controlled his response. *Be casual at all cost; don't look nervous.* The bile in his guts was exploding, yet Jeremiah smiled and with a measured voice replied, "I know. I've been looking for a friend for the last half-hour; I need to find her and take her home. I thought I saw her in front of the store over there, so I made a quick turn. I'm sorry. I know it's not wise to make a U-turn in the middle of the block, but . . . "

"Sir, it is more than not wise; it's illegal. May I see your driver's license?"

Jeremiah reached his right hand into his rear pocket. As he leaned forward in the cab, he reached for the door latch with his left hand to get out of the pickup.

"Sir, please remain in your vehicle."

Jeremiah settled back and took out his license from his leather wallet. The police officer took the license and excused himself. Jeremiah knew the procedure too well. The cop would punch his license number into the mobile computer, and up would flash Jeremiah's driving record. No big deal. It was a false name, but so what? He had gone through a professional to get the proper ID, license and false identity. He had a sterling driving record. Relax.

He couldn't relax.

The young police officer did punch in the numbers, and they came up standard. The guy in the pickup had a clean record. It took all of three minutes for the young policeman to determine the status of the driver; it was what followed on the registration of the vehicle that caught the young officer's attention. The small computer monitor tucked under the patrol car's dashboard displayed a registration breakdown on the pickup. It was registered in Wyoming by a Maryland corporation. The address of the registered owner seemed to be in order; then a Wyoming address appeared. The officer recognized the location immediately as that of the Gateway compound outside of town. Something was gnawing at his thoughts as he looked up at the pickup in front of his patrol car. He leaned over, lowered the right window, and shouted to his partner, who had kept his eyes on the pickup throughout the proceedings.

"Hey, Frank. I remember the chief said something about keeping our eyes open for vehicles coming in from the Gateway compound. What did he want us to do?"

"I don't know. Why not call in and ask the dispatcher?"

"Okay, but what would she know?"

"Just do it."

The dispatcher, a female with a high-pitched voice, told him what he already knew. She knew nothing about what the chief had instructed the officers to do while on patrol. She said she would ask the officer on the desk.

"Frank, I told you she knew nothing." He held up his hands in frustration.

The wait seemed endless for Jeremiah. The young cop should have been back to the pickup handing him a ticket by now. It didn't take all that long in New York to write up a standard moving violation. What was going on?

The chief happened to be at his desk. It was late for him to be at the station, but some exciting things with Martha had kept him there. He had received word from the sheriff's office that they had a statement from a young man who said his buddy had been murdered in the compound. Now the dispatcher told him that Officer Corcoran had pulled over a guy in a pickup from the compound and wanted to know what he should do.

The chief knew exactly what to do. He and Sheriff Harmon had agreed an hour ago that anyone from Gateway should be detained and escorted to the station for questioning.

"Tell him to bring him in . . . and to be careful. We don't know what this fellow may do. Tell 'em to handle him as a dangerous suspect and to search him first; then place him in the secure rear seat of their patrol car."

The dispatcher conveyed the instructions to Corcoran. Then she asked, "Where are you?"

The officer gave his exact location downtown.

"We'll have two backup units there within three minutes, so stay in your patrol car until they arrive. Be careful!"

Officer Corcoran felt the surge of the excitement of a bust, yet there was the anxiety of tracking a wounded tiger in the brush. This was what made all the hours, boring hours, of patrolling pay off in spades. Man, he had a live one at last, something bigger than breaking up a drunken fight in town.

Jeremiah saw the two additional patrol cars bear down on the pickup with red and blue flashing strobes, but no sound of a siren. A crowd began to gather.

They had him blocked. The cop had called for reinforcements. *Damn!* He had suspected something when the ticket didn't materialize. Jeremiah's brain scrambled, trying to compute a plan of action. Should he allow them to arrest him, fingerprint him, check him out, and end up on death row, or go for the assault weapon he had snapped in behind the left bucket seat? It would take all of three seconds to retrieve the gun. He kept it loaded at all times. It would release enough rounds in ten seconds to blast every cop in sight. Jeremiah decided to go for broke. He turned and leaned far enough to his side to touch the butt of the assault rifle. He had to use both hands to release the clips that secured the weapon to the rear of the seat. Even as he fumbled with the latches, he knew he was too late. He had locked the doors, but the two-hundred-fifty-pound officer who came up alongside the pickup from the rear, hugging the truck's bed as he stepped to the driver's side door, glanced in. He saw the butt of the weapon Jeremiah was trying to release.

The officer instantly leveled his shotgun at the window and in a loud voice that could be heard halfway up the block shouted, "Sir, step out of the vehicle. You are under arrest." There was a good deal of emphasis in his voice.

Extreme frustration seized Jeremiah. What to do?

The mesmerized crowd that had gathered began to back away from the scene as more law enforcement vehicles rushed into the block, red and blue strobes twirling atop the patrol vehicles. An officer in the third vehicle, a Dodge Ram, stood on the running board of his vehicle, and in a voice that carried above the sounds of people and engines, gave commands. Another officer emerged from his patrol car and shouted for everyone to get back. Most complied with his orders.

Desperate inside the pickup, Jeremiah fumbled to unlatch the clips that held the weapon secure as a second officer appeared at the passenger side of the pickup with a pistol snubbed against the glass, pointing it at Jeremiah's head. The assassin could see the grim faces outside the pickup. All were poised for his next move. Jeremiah knew he could do immense damage if he began shooting, but he also knew he would be a dead man. The synapses of his brain whirled, trying to sort sense from confusion, but no satisfactory answer came to him. A flow of expletives streamed from Jeremiah's mouth.

He fixed his eyes on the cop at the driver's side of the pickup. The two played the game of ocular chicken. Still the stinging question remained, *What should I do?*

The cop shouted, "Unlock the door, place your hands on your head, and step out of the vehicle. Do you read me?" He repeated the demand, "Unlock the door, NOW!"

The young officer who had initiated the arrest had jumped onto the bed of Jeremiah's pickup and leveled his 12-gauge at Jeremiah's head from the rear sliding window.

With three weapons trained on him, Jeremiah knew he had two choices: He could continue to release the assault weapon and take the blasts that would surely come to the head, and that would end it; or he could comply with their demands and live on death row. What to do?

"Did you understand me? Do as you are told, or we will be forced to remove you from the vehicle." The voice was all business. Time was running out.

The desire for life—any sort of life—prevailed.

Besides, Jeremiah had some pretty incriminating information on the Oracle. It might be worth something as a bargaining chip. With a flicker of his eyelids, he hit the door-lock release, slowly put his hands on his head, and watched as the doors swung open. The burly, young officer on the driver's side reached in, grabbed Jeremiah's jacket by the collar and pulled him from the cab like a tackle grabbing a quarterback in a sack.

It was all over. Jeremiah shook his head like he hadn't a clue as to why they were arresting him, but inside he was filled with bitter frustration.

It was over.

# Chapter 22

Reuben held his head between his hands, his elbows on the edge of the Oracle's desk. Neither Reuben nor the Oracle had uttered a word for the past five minutes. They had reviewed all options for a clean escape from the compound. There were none.

The Oracle whirled about in his leather desk chair to stare out the window once more at the atrium's blank gray wall of bricks and winter-struck plants. He was only conscious of his despair, his anger and frustration. How could his God allow the plans for a Utopian world to crumble like this?

Though he knew that the police had arrested Jeremiah (Security in the cave had picked up the police band and eavesdropped on the reports coming in), the Oracle's mind refused to accept that fact on face value. Jeremiah was too wily to be trapped like that. If he had been caught, then he must have wanted it that way. Sylvia—Mother Martha—would do her plea-bargain thing if they had her as well. He felt certain she had been arrested by now. The Oracle knew that Jeremiah would implicate him in an effort to save himself from death row. It was his bargaining chip. Of course he would use it. Scum like Jeremiah would prefer life in prison to execution. Not so with him.

It had all crumbled so quickly, like an elaborate creation of dominoes. Why hadn't he realized that these two—the two he thought were so loyal—would fall first? Hadn't he personally orchestrated this whole creative venture, paid megabucks for loyalty? And now to be betrayed seemed entirely unexpected, or was it?

Gradually, the Oracle's eyes narrowed, and his mouth twisted into a smirk as he thought of the federal and local authorities lining up their lawmen outside the main gate. He knew they were fully armed, ready to attack given the word from Washington. Did they really think he would surrender? No. If they wanted him, they would have to come and get him. What did he have to gain if he were to surrender?

* * *

The FBI had insisted that all media and worried family members who had gathered stay well beyond the perimeter tape they had strung up outside Gateway. Stephen, Anney, Thom, Samuel and Katherine stood by Stephen's Jeep, which he had pulled up as close to the gate as the barricade allowed. The media could get no closer, but their telescopic lenses brought the main gate clearly into focus for them. In the silence of the standoff the garbled voices of the FBI agents carried as far back as Stephen's and his group. It was hard to understand the words. Hearing was difficult, but viewing through glasses was not. The group watched the action through a couple of binoculars passed around.

They had catnapped through the night at the Jackson Main Motel. Then the sheriff had called them at five that morning to alert them that the FBI had taken over the case, and that with the help of local law enforcement personnel they planned to move in on the compound later in the day. Word had already leaked to the media, so it was no secret. There would be agents streaming in from throughout the West and Midwest all morning. The sheriff had advised that Stephen and the others remain in town, to let the FBI handle it. They refused. Brenda, he knew, was at risk.

It was late afternoon and cold, but not as cold as it had been. The wind that had chilled the group an hour earlier had abated, but even inside her ski jacket and warm pants, Anney was frozen to the bone, more from fear and anxiety than from the frigid weather. Periodically, one or another of the group would slip into the Jeep to warm up. It was Anney's and Stephen's turn again. Todd and Max had left the group behind and were as close to the sheriff's line as possible.

* * *

The Oracle was jarred out of his reverie by the blaring announcement coming from the FBI loudspeaker:

ATTENTION ALL YOU PERSONS INSIDE GATEWAY! WE HAVE BEEN ISSUED A WARRANT TO ENTER YOUR PREMISES. UNLOCK YOUR GATE AND PROCEED OUT OF YOUR COMPOUND IN AN ORDERLY MANNER . . . ! NOW! WE ARE ACTING UNDER THE

AUTHORITY OF THE UNITED STATES GOVERNMENT. NO ONE WILL
BE HARMED IF YOU SURRENDER AS INSTRUCTED.

The announcement was repeated four times. The Oracle scoffed at the
command, quickly contacting his youthful guards at the gate to warn them that
if they opened the gate, they would be shot.

He turned and looked at Reuben, who had lost all color in his face. He sent
him a withering glance. *Look at him, my chief of security, trembling with fear.
They're all traitors. Well, I don't need them anymore.*

The Oracle ignored the voice of  law and order outside the gate. He
suddenly stalked from his office, into the alcove, and down the stairs that led
to the underground passage to the cave. It took him several minutes to walk
from the main structure to the communications center in the heart of the cave.
The brightly lighted center was deserted. Everywhere he turned in the cavern
he felt the emptiness. Always there had been bustle and life within the
mountain. Stillness began to creep under his skin and affect his powers of
reasoning. There was little left to do but make his stand with the authorities.

He retrieved a small key clip from his pocket, then inserted the key inside
the lock on the lid of a small electronic unit next to the surveillance panel. He
opened the lid and read the numbers that had been posted on a strip of  tape at
the base of the unit. Deliberately, he punched in those numbers, hesitating only
a moment before pressing the red "Enter" button which would activate a
detonator that would send a charge to hundreds of pounds of explosives stashed
in strategic areas of the cave. The detonator's timer had been pre-programmed
to send the charge no sooner than thirty minutes from the time it was activated.
The Oracle knew that once activated the timer could be stopped, but one would
have to know the code to halt it. Only he had the code and he had no intention
of halting the timing mechanism that would transform the cave into rubble. He
looked carefully at the minutes remaining on the display, closed the cover,
locked it, then put the key securely back into his front pocket.

While still inside the cave, the Oracle hurriedly strapped eight pin-release
grenades inside an O.D. field jacket and put it on. He had to shift the cumber-
some load as he zipped the jacket up. He then picked up two remaining
grenades and held one in each hand. For yet a moment he studied the small,
flashing, red light on the panel and knew with satisfaction that it signaled an
activated detonator. He opened the door and let himself out of the communica-

tions room and into the hall where he moved with great strides toward the exit tunnel that would return him to his office in the main building.

Nathan, the giant of a young man who spent most of his waking hours in the center, had used the rest room and was returning to the communications room to resume his surveillance of the monitors. With increasing concern, he had been watching the scene outside the compound where the federal agents took up positions to storm Gateway. He knew things were going badly for the Oracle. *How could he help?*

He caught a glimpse of the Oracle as the leader hurried for the tunnel. His first impulse was to shout after the Oracle as he sped away from Nathan toward the exit. He wanted to get an update from his leader about the siege unfolding outside the compound, but he was already through the exit door. Nathan decided not to disturb such an important man. He knew from experience that the Oracle could be brutal in his chiding of those who interfered with his movements. Nathan simply reentered the communications room and sat down in his desk chair where he propped himself in front of the five monitors that scanned the compound in full color.

The Oracle failed to see Nathan as he rushed from the communications room to the exit. He continued across the cave, descended the stairs to the steel door that opened into the passageway and retraced his steps back to the alcove where Reuben had not moved from his chair in front of the desk.

Reuben, the man of steel, the one person the Oracle had relied on to keep order and discipline in the compound, sat confused. All he could pull to the surface of his consciousness was some method of escape. For the several years that Reuben had given his soul to the Oracle, he had never really anticipated this moment of personal crisis. The compound—at least the cave—seemed to him impregnable. But was it? Doubt crowded out all other reasoning for a moment.

It startled Reuben to see the explosives in the Oracle's hands when the leader emerged from the alcove and headed for the hall. He leaped from his chair and shouted, "Where are you going? What in hell do you think you can do to that army with a couple of grenades? Why grenades? We have an arsenal of weapons: missiles, explosives, . . ."

The Oracle did not so much as glance at Reuben. It was as if he were in his own world, a fantasy world, oblivious to his surroundings as he hurried past. Reuben followed. The Oracle stalked through the foyer and out onto the frozen expanse of what had been green lawn a month ago. Now the snow-covered area separated the main building from the main gate by a hundred yards. It was an open space with a frozen pond in the center.

The Oracle moved around the edge of the pond, crunching the hard snow under his boots. Reuben soon came abreast of him, running almost sideways. Beyond the pond, he dashed in front of the Oracle and grabbed him by his sagging field jacket. Reuben felt the grenades lining the inside of the field jacket. His lips began moving before sound emitted. The frosty air turned his breath into white puffs like tiny smoke signals. "Listen, dammit," Reuben yelled in his face, "I want to know what you're planning. I'm in this thing with you. You have to tell me. Where are you going? Tell me what's going on! You have to tell me!"

With his eyes fixed on the main gate, the Oracle pushed Reuben hard to one side as if he were a blocker for the Forty-niners. The hard shove caused Reuben to lose his footing on the slippery snow. He lurched backward, falling to his knees. As quickly as he went down, he scrambled to his feet. However, the Oracle was already ten feet ahead with his hands in front of him. When he reached the metal door of the guard house adjacent to the main gate, he used the grenades as small ramrods. Amazingly, they withstood the impact of his brute force, pounding open the door where he barked at the guards to open the main gate.

The guards were riveted to the TV monitor. Their young heads jerked up at the Oracle's command. "Did you hear me? Open the gate!" he repeated with venom in his demands.

Startled nearly out of his wits, the young guard in command took quick stock of what the Oracle was shouting and said, "What? ... Oh, it's you, sir. .... Yes, sir." With no more thought, he reached across his partner and placed his hands on the computer keyboard. Fidgety and unsure of his abilities, he tried to punch in the code and failed the first time. The Oracle had no patience. He shouted at the top of his voice for the guard to open the gate. The young man, nervous but somehow gaining control, punched in the proper code numbers and waited for the massive gate to slowly retract into the wall. As it did, the gaping passageway revealed a small army of law enforcement officers waiting at a safe distance for just such an action.

As the metal gate slid open, Reuben reached the door to the guardhouse and tried again to halt whatever it was the Oracle seemed to be planning. He shouted, "Stop! Are you crazy?" He thrust his finger at the command guard. "You, reverse the gate. Close it! Close it tight! This is insane."

The word "insane" stopped the Oracle long enough to study Reuben for a split second. He stared at his chief of security, raw hatred filling his eyes. Then, with a powerful lunge, he smashed one of the heavy grenades against the side of Reuben's head. Blood spurted from behind the security chief's ear. The blow slammed him against the metal doorjamb, hitting his head on the opposite side. The Grand Oracle Josiah scorned his security chief and the young guard by declaring, "I'm going to meet my enemy, you cowards."

Pines and alders lined the narrow road leading up to the compound gate twenty feet from where Stephen and Anney were standing. A forest of pines extended back from the road, making a small, tree-covered cove where the hills sloped down to the pines. It had been Anney's suggestion to Stephen that the group go into the secluded little forest and offer a prayer. "Do you remember? We all prayed while we were in that storm on Katherine's ship. We got results. I think we all need to ask the Lord for help now. It would just take a minute."

"Here?" Stephen had asked, looking around at the journalists and law enforcement officers nearby.

"Here or anywhere. Does it matter?" Anney said.

Stephen continued to study the terrain. He turned a full one hundred and eighty degrees and spotted the pine trees. "You're right. We need to offer a prayer again. Let's get the group and head for those trees. Okay?"

Everyone in the Thorns' group followed Stephen into the woods. He offered a brief prayer on behalf of the group. His entire soul seemed to be engulfed in the pleading. For some reason he was not concerned that perhaps it was not in strict conformity to any set order. He simply addressed the Father, reasoned with him, expressed his great love for Brenda, and pled that the Father would lead her to safety.

During the prayer Anney, with tear-filled eyes, glanced up from where she stood in the circle and thought how strong and noble Stephen had become. He had the demeanor of a man of God and shouldered it well. With the "amens" came hugs; then as quickly as they had retreated to the trees, they emerged to their original small knoll where they could continue their vigil. Everyone sensed that something would happen, some event would erupt that would alter this standoff. It soon burst upon them.

The gate was wide open, ready for his exit. With shoulders erect, the Oracle walked defiantly through the opening and ten yards beyond, where he froze, studying the silent crowd of armed men. He glanced beyond the men with rifles at the ready to a more distant group of what he knew to be civilians. They had come to see the show. He would not disappoint them. A twisted smile of satisfaction gradually revealed itself across the lined, gray face. *Yes, . . . it is time. And a fitting audience at that.*

"What's happening, Stephen? What do you see?" Anney's clenched teeth were chattering in sheer terror. She could see without field glasses that the gates had opened, but she was too far away to make out the figure that emerged from the open gate. Through the seemingly endless ordeal, she had learned the true meaning of praying unceasingly. Her whole mind and body surged with faith that her beloved Brenda was safe somewhere beyond the opening to the compound.

"Somebody's coming out," Stephen replied quietly.

"Who is it?"

"A gray-haired man in an army field jacket."

"Do you know who it is, Thom?" Stephen asked. Thom was ten feet in front of the group, wishing he were within ten feet of the guy in the field jacket. He backed up toward Stephen, keeping his raw eyes on the stoic figure outside the opening who seemed as still and immovable as a tree.

Thom took Stephen's field glasses, adjusted them to his vision, and studied the figure at the gate. "I can't get a clear view of the face, but . . . wait . . . it might be the old man himself. I think it is."

"You mean the Oracle?" Anney asked.

"Yeah. I think I'm right. He doesn't have his hands up. . . . Now he's raising his arms out like he was about to surrender. I don't have the foggiest idea what he's up . . . Now he's raising his arms up and out from his shoulders, like he's about to take a swan dive."

Anney reached for Samuel's field glasses . "Please, Samuel, I have to take a look at that monster.

Hearing her request, Burton started to pull the leather strap from over his head and let Anney have his glasses when he noticed that Samuel was handing her his. He quickly turned back to the scene at the gate of the compound, put the glasses to his eyes, and watched, not wanting to miss one moment of the curious happenings unfolding before him. "Is it going to be this simple?" Burton mused, more to himself than to the group huddled a hundred yards from the entrance.

Anney twisted the dial on the field glasses like an impatient child, desperate to adjust them. She was anxious for a close look at the man who had caused her so much grief. Just how evil would this Oracle appear? Soon she was able to focus the glasses and the leader of Gateway came into full view. Anney was surprised as she studied his features. The resolution at a hundred yards was not as clear as she might have hoped, but she could see the high cheek bones and thin face of a man that, strange as it seemed, looked a little like her own father, the Reverend Moore. He appeared to be about the same age as her father. He was thinner in the face, but still he had that look of authority and steadiness that, at times, she had associated with her father. Funny, this man didn't look evil. Anney kept a tight grip on the glasses as she spoke to her husband, "Stephen, he looks a little like Dad."

"What?" Stephen asked, startled that Anney would make the comparison. He studied the Oracle, then commented, "I don't see that."

"What's he doing?" Stephen asked, wanting the glasses back. Burton handed his over. As he did so, he shrugged and said, "I have no idea what he's going to do. He's standing there with his arms outstretched, still as a stork."

The loudspeaker crackled as a new message was issued to the Oracle. Those in command surmised that the man who had emerged from within the compound was the Grand Oracle. They had studied photos of him and were sure it was the key man himself. Again the law enforcement officer shouted through the bullhorn,

"SIR, LIE DOWN ON THE GROUND AND PUT YOUR HANDS BEHIND YOUR BACK."

The order was repeated three times. Everyone in the vicinity clearly heard the instructions that reverberated off the narrow canyon walls.

The Oracle remained immobile. Anney handed Samuel's field glasses over to Thom after she had studied the figure at the entrance long enough to fix his face in her mind. Thom wanted yet another, closer view of what the Oracle was doing.

Again they heard the amplified voice of an FBI agent, repeating the same instructions. Still, the Oracle stood as if frozen in place. It was the sort of moment the FBI men had been trained to anticipate, experience telling them that something surprising could result. They had been trained to make no sudden movements with what could be a hostile subject. Be patient was the word. They had been drilled in patience, even more so since Waco.

One minute, two minutes dragged by. Then, as Stephen squinted into the glasses, there erupted from the spot where the Oracle was standing a bright flash, followed by a cloud of smoke and a powerful blast. The group was caught off guard. As the smoke gradually drifted away, shocked gasps could be heard again and again.

Stephen remembered watching an Indy racer plow into a wall, ripping the car apart. He remembered seeing the driver enveloped in metal and fire. It seemed to happen in slow motion—not unlike this very scene of horror.

Like the smoke itself, the Oracle had disintegrated. Stephen stood stunned. He dropped the glasses to his chest where they dangled by their leather straps. He wanted to get a panoramic view with his naked eyes. All he could see, even at a distance, was that an explosion had removed the Oracle from existence. Except for the quiet gasps of disbelief, the crowd was silent. No one could be certain of what they had witnessed.

Burton spoke first. "He blew himself up!" he said in dismay. He, too, slowly lowered his binoculars. "He did it to himself. No one fired on him. He had explosives strapped to his body."

"How do you know?" Stephen asked.

"I know. He had explosives on him."

Turning a shocked face to Samuel, he repeated, "He blew himself up! I can't believe it. He blew himself to pieces."

Shocking as it was, all Anney could think of was Brenda. "What about Brenda?" she cried, ready to bolt. Stephen sensed this and took hold of her upper arm. He would not allow her to go in, not yet. Who knew what lay in store?

* * *

Always aware that he was a newsman, Burton left the group and rushed forward through the snow to the yellow tape that had been stretched out across the road and up the cliffs on either side to stop all unauthorized persons from going beyond the line of safety. He lifted the yellow plastic tape, bent down, and slipped under it. The young deputy who was posted beside the barricade to prevent anyone from going beyond that point stood as if transfixed, peering through his field glasses at the remains of the Oracle, whose body parts had splattered in a radius of twenty-five or more feet. He was unaware that Burton had slipped under the yellow tape and pushed his way through the officers to the sheriff who stood beside the FBI director.

He said quietly, "Sir, may I go in with you?"

Startled by the voice in his ear, the sheriff turned quickly to see Thom begging for the chance to get what he assumed to be an exclusive. The sheriff studied Burton's face for a moment, then looked behind him down the road to make certain his deputy was in place, then back to Burton. He breathed heavily before he spoke. "Mr. Burton, we don't know when we are going in. But when we do, it's okay with me. But watch your back."

"We're going in pretty quick," said Massey, overhearing the exchange. "The Oracle just blew himself to hell. Pray God we don't run into heavy fire."

# Chapter 23

Nathan watched in stark disbelief as the Oracle destroyed himself. The monitor in the communications center picked up the tragic suicide in full color. The camera perched above the gate continued to film the grotesque scene. It took at least a minute for Nathan to compute what he had witnessed. *The Oracle gone? How can this be? Where does this leave me with all those Feds out there?*

Unnoticed, the timed detonator in the communications center reached the twenty-minute zone on its clock. With twenty minutes remaining to detonation, the timer triggered a mechanism built into the system, setting off a shrill alarm that blasted a sixty-second warning.

The ear-piercing sound brought Nathan to his feet, interrupting his concentration on the monitors. Puzzled for the moment, he glanced in the direction of the sound. He had heard Jeremiah talk about an alarm connected to the Gateway security system. He had never heard the sound, but he was sophisticated enough with electronic equipment to know that it was a warning. A warning for what?

Frantically, he pushed his rolling desk chair out from under him, then took two giant steps toward the master console. Suddenly, it dawned on him. Jeremiah had told him that the cave was wired for explosives —explosives that would provide a final solution should it be necessary to terminate the project. Nathan had no clue as to where the actual explosives were hidden, but he understood that the detonator was on a timer and that undoubtedly the clock was running. On the panel a tiny, bright red light flashed its warning. Below the red light in green LED lettering it read: nineteen minutes, forty-five seconds. Nathan realized in an instant that the Oracle must have come to the cave and set the detonator to trigger an explosion. He had no idea how extensive the range of the blast would be. Would it destroy the whole compound or only the cave? For a moment Nathan tried to figure out how to deprogram the detonator and stop the countdown. But he had no manual and no time to waste. Looking down at the readout, he was certain that within the next few minutes he had to warn everybody to clear out of Gateway. He raced down the hall toward the exit, then stopped. The girls! He couldn't leave those three girls in the cave. He would have to help them get out.

Nathan tore into the therapy hall and found that the three inductees were locked in their rooms. The doors opened from the outside, so he hurried into each of the rooms and shouted at the girls to get out of the building and into the passageway to the main building. Nathan had seen Brenda at least a dozen times in the past few weeks; each time he saw her, he had grown more interested in her. He herded the other two girls down the hall, then spun around to look for Brenda. No sign of her. He rushed back to Brenda's room and found her still lying on her bed, obviously in a drugged state. She seemed unaware of the commotion around her. He scooped her into his arms and carried her out of the room and along the hall of the prefab building to the locked entrance where the other partially sedated girls stood in a daze. The upper part of the door was made of thick, green safety glass. Shouting for the other girls to stand back, Nathan quickly slipped Brenda to the tile floor, leaped into the air, and smashed his boot against the glass, shattering it into a thousand tiny chunks. He reached through the open space and turned the knob; he then picked up Brenda, and nodding toward the two other girls, he moved his charges across the cave and down the stairs, pushed open the heavy steel-reinforced door to the cave, and entered the passageway.

The passageway from the cave to the main building wound underground for a hundred yards. With the confused girls to drag along, it seemed to Nathan as if he were moving a mountain. Finally, he let Brenda's feet slip to the floor. Then he used one arm to support her, leaving the other free to prod the other two along. As the four slowly moved through the passageway, Brenda's bare feet scraped against rough concrete. Her big toe was bent backward, and blood oozed from around the toenail.

"Come on, girls," Nathan shouted in frustration. "Stand up! Walk! You can make it."

At that moment, Reuben loomed in front of the four on his way through the passage to the cave. "Get out of my way! What are you doing in here, anyway?" Reuben barked.

Unaware of Reuben's motives, Nathan was relieved to see the security chief. "Good," he shouted. "I need a strong arm."

"What are you talking about? Get out of my way." Reuben reached out with his hand and pushed Brenda in the ribs to make room to pass. She groaned a weak, painful moan as Reuben shoved past her.

"Hey, man, watch the fist. You hurt her. Why don't you help us?"

"I'm not helping anyone. Get out of my way, I said." Reuben elbowed and shoved his overweight body past the struggling group.

Nathan shouted after the retreating security chief, but Reuben ignored him. He would have told Reuben about the detonator ready to go off, but there was no time to go after him.

Reuben didn't know about the ticking detonator. He was still in shock and bent on escape. Wishing he was twenty pounds lighter, he strained to run as fast as possible along the narrow passageway to the steel door. Reaching it at last, he bolted the door behind him, then he turned to the wall and opened a small fuse-like box and punched in a code. He could hear his heart beating. No one had ever activated the tunnel crusher. As he scrambled up the stairs, he heard the rumbling sound of earth filling up the passageway he had just traversed. The heavy door that divided him from the crushing dirt and rocks held. Reuben could see in his mind's eye the rocks and gravel on the other side of the door extending for seventy yards back along the passageway, making it impossible for anyone to follow him to that point. It had been planned this way by the Oracle to halt any chase by intruders—though it was to have been for the Oracle's escape, not one of his hirelings.

\* \* \*

The roar of the disintegrating passageway came at Nathan and the three girls with the force of a bomb. Nathan's first response was self preservation. He dropped Brenda to the concrete floor in a heap and ran, climbing halfway to the top of the stairs that led to the Oracle's office, dust whirling about him. Then he stopped abruptly. *What am I doing leaving those girls behind? I have to help them. They could never make it up the stairs and out of the building on their own.*

Nathan ran back down the stairs toward the girls. He knew he had wasted at least two vital minutes. How much more time did he have? Seven or eight minutes at the outside? Could he drag three girls up the stairs, through the alcove, sound a warning to the others, and get out the gate before the explosion? He had to grab, push, scream at the girls, whatever, but he *had* to get them to ground level and out beyond the gate. With sheer power that would have been enough to lift a small Geo, Nathan hoisted Brenda back to a standing position and screamed at the other two girls, who were standing once again, "Let's get out of here. NOW!"

* * *

Thom followed Massey and the sheriff as they began to storm the compound. They knew it was risky. When they reached the main gate, they saw hordes of young people pouring from the main building, panic on their faces. Some were running, others walking as quickly as possible. They were all headed for the main entrance, some running barefooted in the snow.

"What's happening?" Thom shouted as he watched the crowd pushing toward them. "They're mighty eager to get out of the place."

Massey warned at the top of his lungs, "Careful. We have no idea what they may do."

Nothing happened. The youths kept coming. The fast ones ran wildly past Burton shouting, "It's going to explode! It going to explode!"

Burton reached out with his long arms and grabbed a young man who tried to rip himself away from him but couldn't. "What's going to explode? Tell me. Do you mean the building is ready to explode?"

"Yeah, the whole place. Let go of me. Nathan warned us a minute ago. Let me go!"

After Nathan had warned the members inside the main building, a couple of fellows who believed him ran to the adjacent facility and alerted the small groups there to evacuate. There were stragglers. Nathan and the three girls limped along, followed by another group of about ten youths.

"I think we'd better fall back," Massey said. "They seem to know something we haven't been told." He yelled for the agent with the bullhorn to shout a retreat to all agents.

"Get back from here, everyone. It may explode!" The agent repeated the warning several times.

By now Stephen had crossed the yellow tape, with Anney right behind him. Frantically he searched among the stragglers for Brenda. *Where is she?* he wondered desperately. Just then he caught sight of a giant of a man half-carrying a limp girl. "It's Brenda!" he shouted over his shoulder to Anney. He ran forward to meet the slow-moving group. Breathless, exhausted to the point of collapse, Nathan refused to let him take Brenda from him, but pushed past him shouting, "Get back! It's not safe here. Hurry. Help us. But move back."

Coming up behind the group, Anney saw Brenda's face exposed in Nathan's arms. She shouted in near hysterics, "Brenda! My Brenda! I'm here, honey! I'm here!"

At that moment the detonator ignited. The explosives placed about the cave exploded, and the earth shook as a loud, muffled explosion rocked the valley. The force threw Anney to the ground. Nathan fell to his knees, still grasping Brenda. Of all the mass of people at the scene, he alone knew the source of the explosion. He knew the cave was now a heap of rubble and that Reuben-- selfish, murderous Reuben, was buried deep inside with a mountain atop him.

Anney crawled the remaining yards to Brenda, who was still dazed. Brenda's face was smeared with dust from the earlier destruction of the passageway. Anney didn't care. This was her little girl. She smothered Brenda's grimy face with kisses and tears. Trembling with shock and emotion, Stephen bent down next to Anney and wrapped his arms around them both.

# Chapter 24

They had left the hospital and sped out of Jackson Hole, relieved that the ordeal was behind them. All had spent the night in their motel, while Brenda lay in a hospital bed in Jackson, undergoing tests. The night before, Burton left with a journalist friend and returned to Salt Lake City to follow up on the biggest story of his journalistic career. Anney and Brenda were in the rear seat of the Cherokee, while Katherine, Max, and Todd rode in Samuel's car. They got away from Jackson by early afternoon and sped over the pass into Idaho.

At first the doctor in charge of Brenda in the hospital was reluctant to release her to her parents. He had to admit that physically Brenda was not severely injured. Emotionally, she was a disaster. It was for this reason she would require immediate medical attention in New Mexico, where she and Anney would arrive after catching their flight from Salt Lake City. Reservations had already been made on a flight to Albuquerque. Stephen had the drive from Jackson scheduled to arrive at the air terminal an hour before departure. At the moment Anney and Brenda were asleep in the rear, and Samuel was speaking softly to Stephen through the open window. Samuel had pulled up behind Stephen's Jeep on the freeway shoulder near Bountiful and had run to the driver's side to confer with Stephen before the two vehicles divided—Stephen, Anney, and Brenda toward the airport, Samuel and his group to Provo. All but the drivers were sleeping. Bone-weary from such intense excitement the past two days, the smooth, rhythmic hum of the highway had induced sleep though it was midafternoon.

"Hope everything goes well for Brenda at Dr. Mucranski's center. It was really good of the doctor to take her so quickly," Samuel said through the open window. Stephen remained behind the steering wheel as Samuel spoke to him.

"Thanks more than I can say, Samuel, for helping out. I don't plan to be home more than a day or so before joining Anney and Brenda in New Mexico. I should be back in Provo in a couple of hours."

From the rear seat Anney stirred, leaning forward behind Stephen's headrest to thank Samuel as well.

"Good luck, Anney," Samuel shouted to be heard over an eighteen-wheeler passing on the freeway. "We'll keep all of you in our prayers. And, Stephen, we'll see you for dinner at Carver's this evening. Okay? 'Bout seven."

"Sure, thanks."

Samuel waved and stepped back as Stephen sent the window electronically to its sealed position, pulled the Jeep's gear into Drive, and sent it back onto the freeway headed down I-215 toward the Salt Lake Airport. Samuel retraced his steps back to his Buick and reported to Katherine, who reclined on the passenger side. Todd and Max in the rear had not stirred from their relaxed position.

* * *

The diffused lighting cast a glow on the heads of the four diners as they chatted amiably. At Samuel's invitation, Dr. Polk had joined the party. The dishes were cleared and the dining room became almost still after the noisy, animated diners meandered out to the parking lot.

At dinner Katherine had lamented that Anney was not with them. She told Stephen that she and Samuel had something special to say. This came after they had recapped what had happened at Gateway.

"Dr. Polk," Samuel began, "coming back in the car, while we were tailing Stephen, Katherine and I got our heads together and came up with something that you may find interesting."

"Sam, you know I'm always interested. What is it?"

"Maybe I'll let Katherine tell you. She is good at such things."

Stephen couldn't help but notice that the overhead lights seemed to illuminate Samuel's head more than the others. It seemed like a halo.

"Samuel," Katherine urged.

"Okay, If Katherine wants me to break the news, I'll do so gladly. As you know, we are getting married. But that is not new." Everyone at the table laughed. They had heard that announcement while the group was still in Jackson Hole. In fact, they had known it was coming sooner or later. "This news concerns the new Book of Mormon Center that is to be built out by Thanksgiving Point. As I said, coming back together, Katherine and I decided to pool our resources —she much more than I—and contribute two million dollars to the project. We see no other way to build the kind of Center all of us want out there."

"Did I hear you right?" A grin shot across Stephen's face, causing deep creases at the corners of his mouth. He glanced at Polk, who was beaming and nodding as if he had known all along.

"Yes, you did," Katherine replied, reaching to touch Stephen's shoulder in a pat of affection and assurance. "The Trust committee, or whatever they call the board, can hardly balk at enlarging the plans with that kind of support from us. And we would like to make the donation in the name of Roy Carver. If you agree, we will select a plaque with Roy's name engraved on it and place it at the entrance to the Center for all to see."

Tears welled up in Polk's eyes. He used his large, linen napkin to wipe them. The very mention of Roy could bring tears, but this on top of the gift was the most touching expression he had heard since Roy's death. He had missed him more than anyone knew.

\* \* \*

Burton walked alongside Dr. Polk's wheelchair as Todd pushed it vigorously along the hall from the elevator to the boardroom. The young man who assisted Dr. Bender had met Samuel's party of six—Katherine and Max included—at the handicapped parking space and escorted them to the boardroom of one of the members, Campbell, who furnished his executive offices.

More alive to the moment than he had been in years, Samuel had looked forward eagerly to this occasion. They had brought into the room extra chairs to accommodate Samuel's guests.

Bender sat down after introducing Samuel and smiled up at him. Katherine sat to Samuel's right. She squeezed his hand as he stood to address the select group.

No stranger to dramatics during a lecture, Samuel began with something interesting and personal to everyone gathered. "I once heard someone say that the Book of Mormon can become to each one of us a personal Urim and Thummim. Think about that. If we were to treat that book as it ought to be treated in our every waking hour, it could be the tool promised us to give us daily guidance." Samuel cleared his throat. "Nephi said something similar when he said this, 'For he that diligently seeketh shall find; and the mysteries of God shall be unfolded unto them by the power of the Holy Ghost.' Now, if that isn't giving us a seer stone to study, I don't know what is."

Samuel continued, "The precious revelations which are in our Book of Mormon, as they fell from the lips of our Savior, are so exquisitely beautiful to me that I cannot imagine anything more marvelous that He could have spoken. Yet, we have the testimony of Mormon that His teachings and revelations to the Nephites went far beyond anything which he had included in his book.

"Mormon called these transcendent precepts 'the greater things' and informed us that he had not written in the Book of Mormon 'even a hundredth part of the teachings of Jesus,' and that he was not allowed to reveal the record to us without first a trial of our faith. In the twenty-sixth chapter of Third Nephi, Mormon offers the greatest spiritual treasure ever made available to mankind. This invitation from God to bestow His richest scriptural gift comes at a price: The cost is full comprehension and belief in His holy record, the Book of Mormon, which the Lord God has sworn that as He lives it is true. Also, there is a penalty attached to spurning this most gracious offering—condemnation! And with this condemnation comes a scourge and judgment. And for taking lightly the proffered holy gift from God, His people have suffered, and may do so again. In short, the condemnation is that the greater things have been withheld from us.

"In light of His revelations, we, His people, must not have fully understood or believed His holy book. If we had, we would have obtained these precious greater things. They were within our grasp at one time. Joseph Smith actually had them in his hands, but had to return them to the Angel Moroni, seal unbroken. It's like having had the most precious jewels in the world in your hands and letting them slip through your fingers because you have failed to do certain rather simple but profound acts to obtain them. What a pity. What was in those marvelous sealed plates that had to be returned? We know part of what was there. For one thing, they contained Christ's teachings that he gave to the Nephites when he taught those surviving people in person. We have got a synopsis of what he taught to those worthy people, but really very little that would make us a Zion Society. Moroni then tells us that the revelations that the premortal Christ gave to the Brother of Jared were also placed in the sealed portion of the plates. And, by the way, those writings of the Brother of Jared were so mighty that they were overpowering for man to read them."

As moderator, Bender felt comfortable interjecting a comment when he asked, "Samuel, tell us what else may have been in those sealed writings."

"Well," Samuel continued, "Moroni gave an invitation to a people that I feel sure are the remnant of Jacob when he said, 'Come unto me, O ye house of Israel, and it shall be made manifest unto you how great things the Father hath laid up for you, from the foundation of the world. . . .' I think this could include Adam's Book of Remembrance and the original writing of the Book of Enoch. Can you imagine what must be sealed up in those writings? I get a thrill up my spine when I think of it. Also, the writings of John mentioned in the Doctrine and Covenants 93 may be there. Think about what we are missing. But Nephi said that the day would come when the sealed book would be read from the house tops . . . and that all things shall be revealed . . . whichever were or ever will be even unto the end of the world. Think of what we have to look forward to!" Samuel inhaled, "It is my opinion that when those marvelous writings are revealed, we will have everything needful to develop a Zion Society and build the New Jerusalem. I would like to pause here for the sake of Sid Bender." Samuel caught Sid's eye and smiled, then said, "Sid, this is the great mystery that no one has caught. The greater things have to be given to the Saints in order for the remaining events to unfold, to create a Zion Society."

Sid pressed his lips together and let his head move up and down. He now understood most of the events that would take place.

Reva Child slightly raised her hand as she spoke. "Then, Brother Meyers, you are saying that we don't have enough revelation to build the New Jerusalem?"

Samuel shook his head. "I think not, for though we were urged and encouraged by the Lord to do this in the revelations in the Doctrine and Covenants, we were unsuccessful in Missouri. We are still living a lesser law when it comes to consecration and unity. Surely, we need those revelations that the Nephites had. They must be like blueprints to living a Zion life and instructions for building the New Jerusalem. But we are without those greater things. We are finishing the sixth millennium, and I think that is significant. Certainly, those events pursuant to the Second Coming must be set into motion before long. If we are not prepared, then what?"

"Another people will be prepared to receive them," Bender blurted out.

"Yes. It was Joseph Smith who warned that if Zion will not purify herself, so as to be approved of in all things—in all things, mind you; not just part, all—then the Lord will seek another people as referred to in this revelation. I'm convinced that the people mentioned will be the remnant of Jacob."

Bender nodded. "Didn't the Lord say that he had consecrated the land of Missouri to the remnant of Jacob, both in His visitation to them shortly after his resurrection, and then to Joseph Smith in the Doctrine and Covenants?"

Samuel leaned forward earnestly. "It appears to me that it will come when the times of the Gentiles are fulfilled and the remnant of Jacob has returned. At that time the remnant will lead out. They will do what we may have failed to do as covenant Gentiles of the Lord. It will likely be they who will bring again Zion, or as the Savior said, those Gentiles who come in unto the covenant will be numbered among the remnant of Jacob and will assist them to build the New Jerusalem.

"Think what we are experiencing and what we have lamentably experienced since the time of the Prophet Joseph Smith and the early Saints."

"What is that?" Moody asked, frowning.

"Unbelief. The Lord has warned us to beware how we hold the oracles of God, which I take to mean prophecies. If we account them as a 'light thing,' then we are brought under condemnation. We will stumble and fall when the storms descend, and the winds blow, and the rains descend and beat upon our house. This happened then and may yet happen in this generation if there is no change. The Lord allowed persecution to storm forth upon the early Saints, both in Missouri and Nauvoo. Did they perceive the cause of so much travail? Probably not. If similar trials happen in our time, will we see the cause? When you consider the extreme effort by the great prophets of the Book of Mormon to get these records to us, and how we tend to esteem the prophecies so lightly, red flags ought to go up. We have to learn more about prophecy and make it part of our very lives. The Book of Mormon, we know, was written for our times."

"What about all of those who are faithful Saints who embrace the Book of Mormon?" Magleby said aloud. "So, what do we need to do?"

"There has to be an outpouring of faith, like nothing we've ever experienced before. Also, there has to be, as I said, a more intense study of prophecy. The Lord wants us to dig deep and know what he has in store for us. We are not doing this as we should. If we had done this, the Land of Zion would have been purchased and redeemed. The law of consecration would have been fully implemented. This accomplished, the Zion Society would have flourished, the New Jerusalem built. It all centers on us obtaining the promised greater scriptures and becoming the salt of the earth. If we had done all this that has been fully spelled out for us by the Lord and His prophets in the scriptures, there would not be only one-sixth of one percent of mankind in His Church today. I think we could have converted vastly more of His children, which would have amounted to hundreds of millions of souls.

"With possession of the greater things, such spiritual and heavenly power would have flowed unto us that none would have had power to hurt His people. If that had been the case, there may even have been no need for Joseph and Hyrum Smith to be martyred. The Lord said to Joseph in Doctrine and Covenants 130, that if he should live to the age of eighty-five, he would have seen the face of the Son of Man. Joseph apparently expected that the New Jerusalem would be built by that time, and that the Lord and the 'powers of heaven' would have come down in their midst.

"Also, if we would believe the Book of Mormon fully and receive the greater things, the news of that would so excite the world that they would fulfill Isaiah's prophecy that ' . . . many people shall go and say'--to their families and friends— 'come ye, and let us go up to the mountain of the Lord, to the house of the God of Jacob; and he will teach us of his ways, and we will walk in his paths . . . '"

"When that day comes, there will be no warring or strife among nations. Through conversion to the gospel, men and women will obey Christ's laws and wickedness will be no more. But let me—"

"Come on, Samuel," Moody interrupted. "Isn't this just a little too idealistic for the real world we live in?"

"The Lord himself has an answer for that. It's in JST Genesis chapter nine, verses 22, 23, He says, *'And this is mine everlasting covenant, that when thy posterity shall embrace the truth, and look upward, then shall Zion look downward, and all the heavens shall shake with gladness, and the earth shall tremble with joy; And the general assembly of the church of the first-born shall come down out of heaven, and possess the earth, and shall have place until the end come. And this is mine everlasting covenant, which I made with thy father Enoch'* "You and I both know the power of the gospel to change the lives of people so that they repent when the truth is given to them. Wonderful things result when people follow the Savior. Still, because of our unyielding stubbornness, those miraculous things that we might have received have been postponed, which, by His foreknowledge, God knew would be the case. Nevertheless, in His justice and mercy, we have been given a full opportunity to have those greater things. The Lord, I'm convinced, will bless this wonderful land—and the remnant of Jacob, his ancient covenant people, will come to the land of Missouri, the Center Stake of Zion. Then those of the Gentiles who have covenanted with our God and continue to abide in those covenants will be made partakers of all the blessings of Zion."

Samuel grew more eloquent than Katherine had ever seen him as she sat at his elbow. He continued, "When this happens, the earth will be renewed and receive her paradisiacal glory, which is to move it into a terrestrial condition with all corruption eliminated. At that stage, He will come and righteousness will cover the earth, 'as the waters cover the sea,' in all of His glory and majesty, and the earth will be filled with the knowledge of the Lord, and His watchmen shall lift up their voice and with the voice together sing this new song."

Samuel then quoted," 'The Lord hath brought again Zion; The Lord hath redeemed his people, Israel, according to the election of grace, which was brought to pass by the faith and covenant of their fathers. The Lord hath redeemed his people, and Satan is bound and time is no longer. The Lord hath gathered all things in one. The Lord hath brought down Zion from above. The Lord hath brought up Zion from beneath. The earth hath travailed and brought forth her strength; And truth is established in her bowels; And the heavens have smiled upon her; And she is clothed with the glory of her God; for he stands in the midst of his people. Glory and honor, and power, and might, be ascribed to our God; For he is full of mercy, justice and grace, and truth, and peace, forever and ever. Amen.'"

Katherine seemed to sense a wonderful spirituality and purity about Samuel as he said with dignity and a prayerful spirit, "Let it be soon, O Lord, that this majestic and glorious hymn shall be set to celestial music. In thy mercy, let us all be found worthy to sing it to thee in the midst of thy Holy City of Zion, and thy great millennial reign be ushered in, that men shall beat their swords into plowshares, and their spears into pruning hooks; that nation shall not lift up the sword against nation; neither shall they learn war any more; that the lion and the lamb shall lie down together, neither shall they hurt nor destroy in all my holy mountain; for the earth shall be full of the knowledge of the Lord, as the waters cover the sea." Samuel lifted his eyes toward the heavens and said, "May these glorious things come to pass, dear Lord, and may we be prepared to participate in them. In the name of Jesus Christ, amen."

Amens echoed throughout the room.

# Chapter 25

Two Gray Lines tour buses idled their diesel engines in the mid-day sun as the drivers waited for their passengers, who were part of the grand opening of the new Book of Mormon Center. It was to become one of their several tourist stops within the radius of Salt Lake City tours. The Center stood fifty yards from the buses and displayed a black glass, pyramid effect. It resembled the Luxor hotel in Las Vegas, shiny, with low plants surrounding it. The grass that spread out from the evergreen plants to the curb was spring green and thick. The entrance had wide, silver, metal-frame, tinted glass doors with large chrome handles. The doors were wide open this noon. Samuel and Katherine had gone through them just moments before to join Stephen and Anney, who had arrived much earlier to be on hand to welcome all the new visitors who were rushing in to take the tour.

On a stone wall eight feet in front of the entrance a bronze plaque had been installed that expressed thanks to the contributors to the Center and further down gave a solemn tribute to Roy Carver. It had been Dr. Polk's desire that the building be dedicated to his memory.

Inside, Samuel and Katherine made their way through the wide foyer and veered off to the side where the Center's offices were situated. The door to the lobby that housed the suite of offices was open and a party seemed to be in full swing inside. In the very center of the roomy reception hall, Dr. Polk sat in his wheelchair shaking hands with a couple that Samuel didn't know.

"Well, Pete, it's a real success," Samuel said, reaching down to touch Polk's hand as he released it from the man before him.

"Oh, Sam. I see you made it. And Katherine."

Katherine also reached out to shake his hand. She looked stunning in her light-blue silk gown and perfectly made up face, hair done in a bun with a slight sparkle. She had dressed for the occasion, which seemed to require an evening dress. She spoke to Dr. Polk a moment. He grasped both of her hands and pumped them, shouting to everyone within hearing distance, "I have to tell all you that this lady and her good husband, Samuel, helped greatly to make this Center possible!"

Heads turned. There were at least three dozen people standing about helping to make the opening of the Center an event. Samuel knew several of the Church General Authorities who had driven down to be part of the celebration. Heads nodded; three couples came forward to meet Samuel and Katherine and express their approval of the project.

"I'm Bill Bennett," Bennett said, then introduced his wife. "I met you, Mr. Meyers, when you accompanied Dr. Polk to one of our committee meetings."

"Yes, yes, " Samuel said. "How are you?"

"Fine . . . May I ask you a question?" Bennett said to Samuel.

"Certainly."

"Dr. Polk tells me that you were present at the announcement of the new location of the Jewish temple in Jerusalem. Have the Jews begun construction?"

Samuel paused a moment, then replied over the hum of the crowd, "Not yet. My Jewish friend who made the announcement assures me that all the material and much of the diplomatic work are in order. I expect that they will begin construction any time now. They have secured the corner stone. It has been washed with sacred water from the pool of Siloam that flows from the Gihon spring, and they anointed it with oil by their Levites and High Priests. All things are in preparation for the start of construction on the temple. It's a great moment to be alive, don't you think?"

"Interesting. I hope it doesn't cause a third world war. I'm not a member of your church, Mr. Meyers, but I do accept the idea that Christ will come to that temple in Jerusalem when He returns."

A guest touched Bennett on the sleeve. He turned to see a friend of his from Phoenix.

Around the room people were smiling and greeting one another. As they spoke, Brenda, with a tray of punch, moved through the gathering, offering anyone that cared a refreshment. Katherine saw her and quickly turned to tap her on the elbow. When Brenda turned around, she seemed to glow with delight. Her face was fuller, skin toned to perfection, hair long and swept back. Katherine sincerely thought Brenda was the most beautiful young lady in the room. She had been to dinner with her and the rest of the family the evening before, but at this moment Katherine was struck anew by Brenda's beauty and charm.

"Honey, you look so . . . so wonderful."

"Thank you, Granny. Care for something?"

"No. I just wanted to look at you. Where is your boy friend?"

"You mean Thom? He's with Daddy, helping with the sound system out in the theater. Isn't it exciting?" Brenda turned slightly to allow an elderly lady with bright, white hair take a cup of punch as she continued to speak to Katherine. "We're getting married, Granny. I told Daddy and Mom about our plans this morning."

"Oh, my sweet, sweet thing. I couldn't be happier for you. I've got to tell Samuel." She reached for his jacket sleeve and began to tug. He interrupted his conversation with Polk, straightened up, and turned to see Brenda.

"Well, well, Brenda—I see they pressed you into service."

Brenda's bright, full-toothed smile reflected her new sincerity toward family.

"Surprise, Samuel," Katherine said with charm. "This young lady just now, very casually, told me she and Thom are getting married."

"That doesn't come as a surprise. I figured you would. He told me at your baptism that he was going to propose to you. I think it's great. You'll make a handsome, smart couple. Have you written to tell Todd?"

"I will this evening."

"How's he doing? I meant to ask last night at dinner." Samuel wanted to know.

"Great. He's a zone leader."

"And his friend . . . ah—"

"Max, honey," Katherine said.

"Max writes Mom and Dad all the time. He's doing great on his mission."

"I'm proud of both of those boys. Katherine and I are going to Osaka in June, and we may get to see Max."

"I hope so, dear," Katherine said, patting Samuel's hand. "Have you decided where you'll be married?"

"If we hold off for two more months, we can both get recommends. I like the new Timpanogos Temple, where you and Samuel got married. Thom likes the traditional old Salt Lake Temple. He thinks it has great Victorian charm. We'll see."

"Brothers and Sisters!" Stephen had entered the room and stood by the doors to make his announcement. "I'm Stephen Thorn and this is my wife, Anney. I'm pleased to be the director of the Center and wish to welcome all of you here today."

The group fell quiet; only two or three continued to finish their comments to one another. Then, in total silence, Stephen spoke. "I want you to know it is a great honor to have you here today as special guests. In a moment we will take the tour. We've had a large crowd all morning, and they are still coming. Even so, we have reserved the noon hour for our special guests—yourselves. Now, then, if you will each line up here at the door, we'll give you the tour of a lifetime. I don't think you will ever experience anything to compare with our gondola ride across Central America, looking down on the small cities that are depicted there. The documented dioramas along the sides of the main arena are very educational as well. Because of time, you will not be able to see everything, nor will you be able to pause long at any one site, but the displays are permanent and you can return any time and gain a greater understanding. Now then, Dr. Polk, would you please bring your wheelchair over here? You will be the first to go on tour."

Polk nodded and began pushing the railing around his wheels toward Stephen. Samuel stepped behind the chair and took over. Everyone seemed elated to be part of the specially arranged tour. Suddenly, Dr. Polk stopped the wheelchair with both hands, tightly squeezing the chrome rims. He looked up to the vaulted ceiling, a broad smile wrapped across his lower face and his eyes shining brighter than they had in years as they watered. He said to those closest, "This is a supreme moment in my life—the fulfillment of a dream. How I wish my good friend Brother Kline were here to enjoy it with me. He would approve. In my wildest imaginings I never thought it would look so splendid."

# References

## Chapter 1
Page 11    • Gathering of the House of Israel—Moses 7:62

## Chapter 3
Page 40    • Adam's history—D&C 107:53-54

## Chapter 7
Page 77    • Nephite's return—3 Nephi 21:1, 20:22, 2 Nephi 10:19; Mormon 3:17; D&C 52:2
     • (Nephites were also called "House of Israel" because they are Israelites.)

Page 79    • John the Revelator among Lost Tribes—H.C., vol. I, pg. 176, 2 Nephi 29:12, 13

## Chapter 10
Page 92    • "Wicked will slay the wicked, and fear shall come upon every man." Times of Gentiles fulfilled—D&C 63:33; D&C 45:30

Page 95    • Gathering—In June 1831 conference, Joseph Smith prophesied that "John the Revelator was then among the Ten Tribes of Israel, who had been led away by Shalmaneser, King of Assyria, to prepare them for their return from their long dispersion, to again possess the land of their fathers."
     • Lamanites first to enter New Jerusalem after it is built—3 Nephi 21:24; D&C 49:24.
     • Moses 7:62-63
     • More part of all the tribes have been led away"—I Nephi 22:4
     • D&C 29:9—"Wickedness shall not be upon the earth."
     • D&C 63:33

## Chapter 11
Page 113    • 2 Nephi 10:19
     • Young lions—3 Nephi 20:16; 21:12
     • 3 Nephi 21:1—establish, begin Zion.
     • Build New Jerusalem - remnant of Jacob and Covenant Gentiles—

3 Nephi 21:22,23

# Chapter 12

# Chapter 24